The Soy Revolution

The Soy Revolution

The Food of the Next Millennium

STEPHEN HOLT, M.D.

M. Evans and Company, Inc.
New York

M. Evans and Company, Inc.
216 East 49th Street
New York, New York 10017

LCCN: 98-073645
ISBN: 0-87131-854-7

Book design and text formatting by Bernard Schleifer
Printed in the United States of America

9 8 7 6 5 4 3 2 1

Contents

Special Note

In this book author Stephen Holt, M.D., provides information that represents his interpretation of soybean research and, in this capacity, is *not* making any medical treatment recommendations or any statements that support disease prevention protocols. The U.S. Dietary Supplement and Health Education of 1994 stipulates that dietary supplements are not to be used to prevent or treat any disease. Similar regulations exist in many other countries. Dr. Holt does not recommend self-medication and encourages individuals to discuss medical treatments, dietary adjustments, or any health-care intervention with a qualified health-care practitioner. *Please do not self-medicate in the face of significant illness.*

Nothing that is communicated in this book should be considered an attempt to recommend nonstandard advice for the prevention or cure of any or all diseases. Certain fractions or components of soybeans contain highly potent compounds with unknown toxicities to humans when consumed in high doses. For example, soy isoflavones (*e.g.*, genistein) are powerful compounds to be used with caution.

No statements in this book have been evaluated by the U.S. Food and Drug Administration or any other regulatory agency. Any products or foods mentioned by the author are not recommended by the author with the intention of diagnosis, treatment, cure, or prevention of any or all diseases.

Foreword

Dr. Stephen Holt has made a major contribution to the research and development of soy foods and dietary supplements made from soy. Part of his commitment has been to engage in extensive educational activity in reporting the role of soy in the prevention and potential treatment of a variety of diseases. Following the publication of *Soya For Health* by Mary Ann Liebert Inc., Larchmont, New York, an explosive interest in the potential health benefits of soy foods and supplements determined the need for Dr. Holt to write this new book, *The Soy Revolution,* so that advances in research can be more widely communicated. Dr. Holt's first book rapidly became a bestseller among health-care givers for whom the book was primarily written. This present work presents a lucid account of exciting developments in soybean research and contains much new information that has surfaced in scientific studies of soy over the past two years.

Some of Dr. Holt's earlier assertions on the potential health benefits of soy have been confirmed in recent clinical trials. These assertions were brave in the face of some residual skepticism about the health-giving effects of the soybean. The book is written in Dr. Holt's usual eloquent style, but he has mastered the difficult task that a scientist faces when he must communicate difficult or incompletely understood interest and it provides an excellent source of concepts, speculations, and reasoning about the health benefits of soy.

During 1997, it was difficult to find a popular magazine that did not run at least one story about the health benefits of soy foods and dietary supplements made from fractions of soy. Some of the information imparted to the general public in these popular periodicals has been incomplete and, on occasion, misleading. Dr. Holt clarifies the important issues of the nutritional value of soy, and he describes the potential benefit of soy in the management of many common diseases in a painstaking manner.

Dr. Holt has worked on nutrition in therapeutics for more than twenty years, and he has devoted much of his professional activity over the past five years to the research and development of soy foods and soy supplements. I believe that this book supersedes all the other general books on the health benefits of soy, and it presents the most up-to-date status report of soy and health for a wide audience of readers. Dr. Holt has walked a tightrope between his accomplishments as a scientist and his role as a thought-leader in the food and dietary supplement industry. His work is objective, and it reflects his enthusiasm for nutritional interventions for disease-state management.

Dr. Holt brings a unique perspective to the food and supplement industry by virtue of his background in clinical and basic science research in therapeutics. He has not supported the health benefits of soy food lightly, and his encyclopedic knowledge of the subject has made him a frequent guest lecturer on the subject of soy at scientific meetings and in the general media.

It is difficult for many to recognize the power of Dr. Holt's work in the soyfood industry, where he has contributed greatly to facilitate communication between the East and the West. Dr. Holt's contributions are enigmatic to some degree. The recognition of his work in soybean research has resulted in frequent invitations to lecture to Asian soy food societies, and he has been appointed to a leading role in the direction, planning, and institution of basic science and clinical research at the Central Research Institute for Soyfood Research in Korea. This institute is funded by Dr. Chai-Won Chung, an octogenarian pediatrician who has made one of the largest contributions to the application of soy food in health care through his famous company that dominates the soy food market in Korea.

To quote Dr. Holt: "Soy food may well be the food of the next millennium." This book presents powerful evidence to support a switch—or even partial move—from animal protein–to vegetable protein–based diets that can incorporate soy for health in the face of Dr. Holt's characterization of the "Soy Revolution."

T.V. Taylor, M.D. FRCS
Professor and Chief of Surgery
Veterans Administration Hospital
Baylor College of Medicine
Houston, Texas

Preface

Nutritional interventions in medical practice to treat or prevent disease is moving away from "mythical" and "magical" thinking. *The Soy Revolution* presents the increasing evidence that dietary adjustments can have a profound influence on the health of humankind. The content of this book is not novel, and in many cases it does not even represent new information. I have taken the work of thousands of researchers in the "soybean field" and reported and/or interpreted their findings. Therefore, it is not possible for me to acknowledge everyone who has contributed to the immense and impressive database that exists on the potential health benefits of soy.

To say that I am impressed by the health-giving potential of soy food or fractions of soy used in well-formulated dietary supplements is an understatement. I have attempted to balance my enthusiasm for the use of soy products to promote health by concentrating on the facts. However, opinions are divided in some areas on the specific actions or health benefits of soy. Still, I believe that a consensus can be garnered to support the "notions" that I present.

I am very involved in the dietary supplement industry and admit a great interest in researching and developing nutritional or botanical interventions that can be used to promote wellness. This leaves some room for individuals to draw attention to my enthusiasm for dietary supplements made from soy, but I reject any implied conflict or contention.

I would like to see the health benefits of soy foods presented in standard dietary format, but the Western palate may not be attuned to many soybean-based foods and, more important, predictable and continuous intake of certain fractions of soybeans is required to achieve the desired health benefits. At the time of this writing, and perhaps for several years to come, soy foods will not be generally available in a format that is engineered to provide the amounts and factions of soy that confer selected health benefits. That is why I believe that dietary supplements made from soy make sense and the reason I have dedicated much of the past five years of my professional activity to developing food supplements and foods from soy that can confer real and measurable health benefits.

Medicine has been described as being at a crossroads when it comes to conventional medical practice and alternative/complementary medical practice. Blending the two disciplines under the umbrella of "integrated medicine" has been proposed, but this approach does little to dispel the existing dichotomy in medicine. Many factors contribute to changes in medical practice, but the interest in alternative medicine and nutritional interventions have been driven by consumers of health care who exhibit a new self-reliance to live longer, be healthier, and look for gentler, more natural alternatives to allopathic (conventional) medicine.

The failure of allopathic medicine to eradicate common killer or maiming diseases such as cardiovascular disease, arthritis, and cancer with drugs or invasive treatments may be described as a premature judgment, but humankind is increasingly impatient to be well. I balance this statement by saying that many disciplines of alternative medicine have yet to convince society of its alleged safety and efficacy in many areas. I despise the labels conventional, alternative, complementary, and integrated because they serve little purpose in an age where we should be preoccupied with what works, not its origins.

Since the publication of my first book on soy, *Soya For Health* (Mary Ann Liebert Publishers, Larchmont, New York, 1995), I have found increasing acceptance of some of my proposals on the demonstrated or putative health benefits of soy. However, some of my colleagues in academic medicine have asked me if I need psychiatric help! There is a danger of being a conventional physician who dares to explore the perceived myths and magic of the nutritional approach to disease. One can end up with no friends if one wants to question the conventional (pharmacological or surgical) approach to disease without embracing the alternative or complementary approach with whole-hearted enthusiasm.

Against this background, I have tested my own version of scientific reality and I have concluded that soy is food of the next millennium. Soy has versatile and powerful health-giving benefits, which has been shown by a lot of credible basic science and clinical research to be unquestionable. As we struggle to manage the unmanageable groups of chronic degenerative diseases that afflict industrialized societies, we must pause and reexamine the cause of these diseases. Chronic diseases that cause excessive suffering (morbidity) and death (mortality) are largely determined by adverse lifestyles. Lifestyle involves moderation in living, exercise, emotional well-being, and good nutrition. Of all the facets of lifestyle that are amenable to rapid adjustment, nutrition stands out. Soy foods are not only good sources of nutrition, they can prevent diseases and, in some cases, fractions of soy can treat diseases.

One may wonder why an author would write two books on soy within a period of three years. *Soya For Health* was written for healthcare givers; it was extensively referenced and, therefore, somewhat staccato in style. Some of the information in my earlier book may be beyond the reach of readers who do not have advanced knowledge of science. This book is geared to everyone who wants a rapid update on areas of interest in soy foods and health, but it is written in a style and format that should appeal to a layperson and, I hope, not bore the well-informed.

I have had a lot of help in toning down my writing by Virginia McCullough, a professional writer who is an expert in editing health care books for general readers. I acknowledge the help and advice received from many people involved in the soy food industry and in nutrition research who have imparted much knowledge to me.

Please read this book in health and allow its contents to transform your life. Please share the concepts that I propose about soy foods and dietary supplements with your health-care providers. This book concentrates on matters of fact, and soy holds the promise of enhancing your health and well-being.

Revolutions are often met with resistance, but when well-planned and carefully enacted, they can be successful. I strongly believe that soy is begging to offer humankind a new way to seek health as we enter the next century.

STEPHEN HOLT, M.D.
President and CEO,
Biotherapies, Inc.
Fairfield, New Jersey
January 1998

The Soy Revolution

CHAPTER 1

"I've Heard About the Benefits of Soy, But..."

Most people are tired of being told that their diet is unhealthy, but they are acutely aware of the importance of nutrition for health. If you are like most consumers today, you are concerned about your health and have probably resolved to improve your diet. You have heard about soybean products, but you may not know exactly what it is that makes them healthful foods, so you are not sure why you should make an effort to include soy-based foods in your diet. This book should help you solve these dilemmas.

Let me assure you that adding soy foods to your diet is not another nutritional fad, nor am I a "soy nut." However, this book does present a significant amount of information about the health benefits of soy and points you toward a natural way to better health.

This book is a synthesis of the main research findings of thousands of dedicated scientists and health-care workers, and it reflects my interpretation of the literature. For readers who require more technical information and referenced resources, this is provided in my first book, *Soya For Health*.

The Soy Revolution also explains what you should know about foods and dietary supplements derived from soybeans. For a variety of reasons, you will be hearing more about soybeans in the coming decade or two and, in fact, I believe the health benefits of the soybean are so important that I described this plant as the "food for the next millennium," during my plenary lecture to the Korean Soyfood Association in Seoul, South Korea, in 1997.

It is no exaggeration to say that new research findings about soy appear, quite literally, every day. A day does not go by without popular news media or the medical press reporting on the newly discovered benefits of components of soy. While I was writing this book, just when I thought the information presented was complete one more important soy study appeared, taking me back to the manuscript to add more material.

Some of the material you will read in this book might seem a bit technical, but there is no way to do justice to the vast amounts of information available without examining in detail the chemical components of a plant that is one of nature's most important nutritional gifts. Bear with me on this; you will find that by the end of the book, you will have information that can change your life.

Research reveals that in the future soy can play an important role in reducing the incidence of many degenerative diseases and illnesses that are the leading causes of death in most Western countries. If people are serious about preventing or treating conditions such as heart disease, hypertension (high blood pressure), cancer, and diabetes, they will need to consider adding soy foods to their diets.

Equally exciting are the potential preventive and healing properties of soy for conditions such as osteoporosis, kidney disease, conditions of the prostate gland, various gastrointestinal disorders, and obesity. Soy also has a part to play in easing the symptoms and adverse health consequences of menopause, maintaining normal weight, and enhancing athletic performance. In addition, I believe that soy may contribute to retarding the aging process. Indeed, preventing the common diseases associated with aging represents a giant leap in improving our quality of life as we grow older. Many people in our culture live into their seventies, eighties, and even their nineties, but spend too many of these later years coping with ill health. I believe that soy can help people feel better and live longer, with an enhanced quality of life.

This book attempts to sort through the facts about soy and guide you to the best ways to use this unique food in order to build and maintain health. You probably know that fractions of soy are used as an additive in many commercial food products and that soy is a viable substitute for animal protein. While it is true that soy is a high-quality protein food, that is just the beginning of the soybean story. Nor are all soy products created equal; each has unique characteristics and strengths. Some processed soy foods also have weaknesses.

In the West, soy is a relatively new addition to the array of foods considered fit for human consumption. Until the last couple of decades, most North Americans and Europeans thought that soy was little more than a plant used to produce soy sauce and animal feed. Then, soy-based milk substitutes and protein drinks were introduced and some "natural" food markets started to sell such products as "soyburgers," which were billed as meat substitutes. Yet most of the several billion bushels of soybeans American farmers produce annually is used as animal feed or is exported. The Japanese and Koreans are two of the biggest customers. People who explore the commodities markets quickly learn that the soybean crop is of critical importance to the agricultural sector of our economy. Soy derivatives are also used in many nonfood commercial products such as adhesives, building materials, and even breast implants. The famous entrepreneur, Henry Ford, once sported a suit made from fabric produced with soybeans!

Though soy is a relatively new food source in the West, it is an ancient one in the East. Soy has been a dietary staple in eastern Asia for more than 3,000 years. To understand the potential significance of soy as a beneficial food for human beings and an ecologically positive crop for our planet too, it is helpful to understand the role that soy has had in other cultures.

THE SACRED PLANT

Soybean cultivation probably originated in northern China and Inner Mongolia before it eventually spread throughout Asia. It is known to have been cultivated in China as early as 4,000 years ago. For many centuries the plant was an important staple food in Korea, Japan, and other Asian countries. The expansion of the Buddhist religion throughout Asia, with its vegetarian philosophy, was an important influence for the adoption of soy as a staple food. Over the centuries Buddhist monks have flavored soy in numerous ways to produce delicious vegetarian meals with soy protein. Some of these dishes have a taste that is indistinguishable from veal or pork.

The Chinese word for soybean is *ta-tou*, which means "greater bean." It was considered so valuable for human (and animal) health, that the Chinese Emperor Shen-Nong declared it one of the five sacred crops. This emperor researched the healing properties of over one hundred plants and compiled the earliest known medical treatise, entitled *The Medical Bible of the Yellow Emperor*.

By the middle of the fifth century CE, soybean foods were used therapeutically in China to restore proper heart, liver, kidney, stomach, and bowel functioning. Ancient Chinese medical writings discuss soy derivatives, most notably in the work of Taoist physician Szu-miao. Known as the "King of Medicaments," Szu-miao practiced at the beginning of the Tang dynasty (early in the eighth century). He identified the various types of soybeans, much modern research confirms what he recorded centuries ago.

In the sixteenth century, during the Ming dynasty, physician Li-Shi-zhen spent more than thirty years compiling a fifty-two volume Chinese *Materia Medica* of pharmaceutical botany in which soybeans are described as effective remedies for such conditions as edema (abnormal water retention), kidney disease, and poisoning. Contemporary researchers also have corroborated the findings of Li-Shi-zhen's sixteenth-century research.

In contemporary China, soy is known as "China cow" because it is used to make soy milk, an excellent alternative to animal milk. Soy milk is a versatile and healthful source of protein that is devoid of saturated fat. As we accept the obvious evidence that soy protein is a healthful alternative to dairy protein, I believe soy milk will one day overtake dairy milk in the Western diet.

Soybeans are hardy crops, and there is no question that cultivating the soybean has allowed the Chinese people—and other Asians—to survive in spite of famines, political and social upheavals, and numerous natural disasters. In addition, the incidence of cardiovascular disease, hypertension, diabetes mellitus, and cancer, when compared with that of Europeans and North Americans, is generally lower among the Asian populations who eat a traditional soy-based diet. We can be grateful that a food considered sacred in one part of the world has finally made its way to our society, even though it has taken many centuries to get here.

SOYBEANS TRAVEL TO THE WEST

One version has it that soybeans first arrived in the United States from China early in the nineteenth century as ballast in a Yankee clipper ship. Others claim soybeans made their way to the U.S. via Europe, perhaps being introduced by the British, who took soybeans from China. However, it took more than another century before soy began to be viewed as a significant food source for humans in either Europe or America.

During World War I there was a shortage of inexpensive oils, both for industrial use and human consumption. Since it is a great source of oil, there was an economic incentive to cultivate the hardy soybean. However, the soybean's true nutritional value was not yet recognized. Throughout the 1920s and '30s, soybeans were considered most valuable for their oil, and soy meal was treated as a mere by-product. Soybean growers were encouraged to develop varieties of soybeans with a high oil content. Because the flavor of the oil was not considered palatable to Americans, the oil was used for industrial purposes. By the end of the 1930s, though, new processing techniques solved the flavor problem, and soy oil began to become important in the food processing industry. Recognition of the value of soy meal for animal feed quickly followed and, after World War II, there was an ever-increasing demand for soy protein products to feed to domestic animals.

In spite of a majority opinion that restricted soybeans to industrial uses, or to being used as animal feed, there were people who saw greater value from this plant. Early in the twentieth century natural health advocate John Harvey Kellogg believed that soy products were useful in treating diabetes mellitus. Dr. Kellogg distinguished his famous Battle Creek Sanitarium and developed cereal food products, including granola, that he hoped would lure the population away from breakfasts of sausage, bacon, and eggs. As an advocate of a vegetarian diet, Dr. Kellogg stood relatively alone during his era and in many ways was ahead of his time.

Vegetarianism has never been widely popular in the United States, but vegetarians became the primary developers of soybean food products. The Seventh-Day Adventists, founded by Ellen G. White in the mid-1880s, promoted a vegetarian diet among its members and became the first North Americans to use soybeans as a staple food product. The concept of creating meat substitutes—called analogs—began when members of this church developed "look-alike" food products that would be palatable to North Americans. Presumably, members of the Seventh-Day Adventist church took the culinary lead from Buddhist monks, who are the masters of making "look-alike" soy foods.

Seventh-Day Adventists currently play an important role in the soy food industry in the United States. It is not surprising that studies of the health status of Seventh-Day Adventists reveal that when compared to others in the U.S. population, they have lower incidence of heart disease, hypertension, and other chronic diseases. This religious sect apparently knows what many others in the West do not: the soybean is a very special plant!

As the soybean plant has "traveled" throughout the world, thousands of varieties and strains have been developed. American farmers, who account for about 40 percent of the world's total soybean crop, grow about forty different varieties. Through genetic engineering, soybean growth can be manipulated to strengthen its individual components. For example, agribusiness giant Archer Daniels Midland (ADM) developed a variety of soybean from which vitamin E supplements are formulated. ADM has done a great deal to promote health in the Western civilization by developing and refining uses for soybeans.

Thus, the soybean is indeed here to stay in the West. During this century, there has been a growing demand for soy products, both for consumption and for industrial use, in such places as Brazil, Argentina, South Africa, and many European countries.

Although there is increasing interest in the nutritional value of soy, the industrial uses are vast and continue to grow. This is nothing new, however. In China, hundreds of years ago, soy oil was used in caulking for boats or as lamp oil for homes and temples. Today, products as diverse as soap and shampoo, antistatic agents, ink, cement, household cleaners, resins, adhesives, and fabric are produced using soy derivatives.

EATING SOY FOR HEALTH

When eaten in a crude form, the soybean is not a friendly food. Anyone who has ever eaten crude soybean knows about the predictable abdominal gurgling, the funny taste or bitter aftertaste, and the embarrassing gas. Without the developments in modern food technology that have made soy foods palatable, soy would not be consumed to any degree in Western society.

The general well-being that can be the reward of eating soy foods comes from their general nutrient content. They are low in saturated fat and provide readily assimilated forms of essential amino acids. Soybeans have a good vitamin profile (A, E, K, and some B vitamins), and they have an excellent balanced mineral content (potassium, iron, phosphorus, and calcium). Of special interest are the plant compounds (phytochemicals) such as isoflavones (genistein and daidzein). These compounds, abundant in soybeans, have special health-giving benefits. Soy isoflavones will be discussed in detail in Chapter 3, and you will notice that their role in maintaining health and preventing disease is raised repeatedly throughout this book.

I clearly recognize that many people with a typical Western lifestyle cannot eat enough soy foods to derive consistent health benefits. Furthermore, some commercial soy foods are not standardized for their health-giving fractions, such as isoflavones. For this reason, many people prefer to receive the health benefits of soy through dietary supplements. These supplements have predictable amounts of the healthful components of soy, and the nutritional supplement format suits a busy adult with a "Western palate." I discuss the advantages of some soy-derived dietary supplements in later sections of this book.

WHAT MAKES SOYBEANS SPECIAL—AND IMPORTANT?

The soybean is among the very few plants that provide a complete protein source. By that I mean that soybeans contain the essential amino acids that form what is known as a *complete protein.* Essential amino acids cannot be synthesized by the body and therefore, must be obtained from food. Some of these amino acids might sound familiar: lysine, tryptophan, leucine, phenylalanine, methionine, histidine, isoleucine, threonine, and valine. Animal protein sources also contain the essential amino acids, for this reason, meat, poultry, fish, eggs, and dairy products have long been considered mainstays of a healthful Western diet.

Soy foods have become widely available in the West at the very time extensive research has confirmed that we need to consume less fat and more fiber. In addition, while protein intake is essential because we require amino acids and nitrogen, most people in Western countries consume more than is needed to build and maintain health. The standard established by the National Research Council serves as a guide. We need about half a gram of protein per kilogram (2.2 pounds) of body weight (ideal body weight, that is). Proteins vary in quality, so, as a precaution, 0.8 grams serves as a guideline to ensure adequate protein consumption. This means that a woman whose ideal weight is 140 pounds (roughly 63.5 kilograms) needs to consume about 51 grams of protein a day. In the West, there is generally no need to count protein grams because this amount of protein is so easily available.

One serving of tuna fish, for example, supplies about 20 grams; a three-ounce hamburger provides about 21 grams; an ounce of cheddar cheese supplies about 14 grams of protein. Assuming that the average person eats some vegetable and grain products, which also contain protein, we can see that the average Westerner consumes more than enough protein. In fact, the average man in the U.S. consumes about 100 grams of protein a day.

It is true that pregnant women, women who are breast-feeding, children, and elite athletes or bodybuilders need more protein than the average adult, but these special needs are generally easily met in our affluent society. Overconsumption of protein is a far greater concern for most people in Western countries. Excessive intake of animal protein in the West has been clearly linked with the development of chronic degenerative diseases and causes of premature death and disability in Western societies.

The harmful consequences of basing a diet on animal proteins comes from the fact that these foods are relatively high in saturated fat and cholesterol, and they contain no fiber at all. For this reason, the typical Western diet is relatively low in fiber when compared to a typical vegetarian diet, which relies on grains, beans, legumes, vegetables, fruits, and nuts to supply protein and fiber in the diet. Since the soybean provides high-quality protein; is relatively low in fat content; includes generous amounts of many vitamins and minerals; and, in many of its consumable forms, contains fiber, this legume is the answer to our "dietary prayers."

PROTEIN MYTHS

Many myths surround the notion that our diets must be based on animal protein. First, we have made the mistaken assumption that meat and other animal foods automatically provide high-quality protein. The percentage of usable protein varies among animal products, while soybeans consistently contain 35 percent protein by volume, most of which is easily used by the body.

When comparing protein content of foods, it is interesting to note that one-quarter pound of meat or poultry contains approximately 18 to 22 grams of protein, and one-half cup of cooked soybeans contains 20 grams. In both cases, the protein is complete in that it supplies all of the essential amino acids. The fat content of four ounces of meat or poultry varies, but we know that animal fats may raise cholesterol levels in the blood and in excess they are not particularly beneficial to humans. Nowadays, health-conscious consumers find ways to cut the fat content of animal protein by removing the skin from chicken, buying the leanest cuts of meat and trimming all the fat, and by using nonfat or reduced fat dairy products. While this certainly helps reduce overall fat intake, some saturated fat still remains; in addition, animal protein and cholesterol consumption remains higher than necessary.

Those who eat a vegetarian diet are usually familiar with the concept of complementary proteins, meaning that they eat two or three different foods, each containing some of the essential amino acids. What one food lacks the other provides. A lunch consisting of lentil soup and cornbread, for example, provides complementary amino acids so a complete protein is formed. A dish made with correctly chosen vegetables and soybeans provides a complete protein; no other food is needed to form a complete protein component in that meal.

In the 1970s, activist and author Frances Moore Lappe published *Diet for a Small Planet*, a book that raised public consciousness about the value of a plant-based diet. Lappe, in trying to explode the myth that humans require animal protein, led readers to believe that they needed to be vigilant about combining proteins in order to insure that a complete protein was obtained in each meal. She correctly pointed out that virtually all societies meet their protein needs by combining foods with differing amino acid content. Meals featuring dishes using beans with nuts, seeds, wheat, corn, or rice, for example, result in a complete protein. However, it is not necessary to be overly concerned about consuming foods with complementary amino acids in every meal. A diet in which most of the calories are consumed from plants generally supplies amino acids adequate to build sufficient protein to meet all our requirements. Of course, a soy-based diet eliminates the concern altogether, since all the essential amino acids are present in soy.

THE RESEARCH EXISTS

When we consider the existing research on the effects of soy, it is inevitably surprising that this legume has not already become a staple of the Western diet. Obviously, change comes slowly, and the economic and social forces supporting meat-based diets have been slow to abandon the idea that animal protein is the centerpiece of a healthful diet. The new food pyramid endorsed by the USDA (U.S. Department of Agriculture) represents a major progressive step in that it recommends that complex carbohydrates—grains, beans, vegetables, nuts, and seeds—form the foundation of the diet and serve as the primary source of our calories. For the first time in this country's history, a government-endorsed diet de-emphasizes animal protein. These new dietary recommendations open the door to embrace soybean products as a primary source of protein.

Long before the new food pyramid was endorsed, however, researchers were discovering the health benefits of soy. Mark Messina, Ph.D., a prominent researcher on the relationship between soy and cancer prevention, organized the First International Symposium on the Role of Soy in Preventing and Treating Chronic Disease. Held in Mesa, Arizona, in 1995, this meeting provided a glimpse of the vast range of health benefits soy products offer. At this first symposium, thirty-four papers were presented on such topics as cholesterol reduction and cancer prevention. By 1996, the movement to study the role of soy in preventing and treating chronic disease was well underway, and Dr. Messina hosted the Second International Symposium, held in the fall of 1996 in Brussels, Belgium. More than seventy papers were presented that highlighted the unquestionable health benefits of soy. Throughout this book I will refer to research that has isolated particular chemical components of soy that prove beneficial for various conditions; while others have investigated possible negative side-effects of soy, to date, no study of humans has shown that soy poses any health risk.

The food industry itself has made contributions to the research on soy, particularly because studies have confirmed that plant-based diets are usually low in fat. Since low-fat diets are associated with lower cholesterol levels and reduced incidence of heart disease, the food industry is quite naturally looking ahead to a time when Westerners turn to efficient, low-cost and low-fat protein food sources. Does this mean that I or other researchers advocate complete vegetarianism? Should we all be throwing out our meat roasters and living on tofu and vegetable stir-fry dishes?

It is not necessary to become a complete vegetarian. Currently, most researchers believe that small but significant changes in the typical American diet will bring positive results. For most of us, drastic dietary changes seldom last very long anyway. It is far better to gradually add soy and other valuable plant proteins to our diets, substituting them for some of the animal protein we normally eat. This will allow us to reap the benefits over time.

THE ENVIRONMENTAL CONNECTION

It is no secret that despite the "Green Revolution" of the last forty or fifty years, we find ourselves in a situation in which food resources are often abundant in some regions and tragically scarce in others. Growing population puts pressure on available arable land in certain areas of the earth. Land that was once used to grow crops falls to the encroaching desert in some countries and encroaching urbanization in others.

Western countries, particularly those with a large land mass and lower population density, have used their agricultural land to support a meat-based diet. This is a luxury we may not be able to afford much longer. In simple terms, what current land-use policy means is that in order to produce vast quantities of beef and other animal foods, we must use land to produce grains that are used solely for animal feed. In other words, the same oats, barley, soybeans, and corn that would be consumed by humans in other parts of the world are being fed to animals, who, in turn, provide our population with expensive sources of complete protein. It is true that beef cattle are efficient protein machines. If we feed them enough soy and other plant proteins, they predictably turn out hamburgers and steak. The trouble is that it takes about seven pounds of grain and soybeans to produce one pound of usable animal protein. This is a conservative estimate; others who have attempted to document this have put the ratio as high as twenty pounds of grain to one pound of resulting protein. So, while the animals might be efficient producers, plant protein derived from the land makes more sense as a basic, cost-effective source of food.

Soybeans hold the answer to one piece of the environmental puzzle, to the extent that an increased demand for protein can be partially met by using this plant. The soybean can be transformed into myriad products, for humans rather than for animals. This means that we in the West will probably need to consume less meat and poultry and more tofu and tempeh. As it happens, this would hardly be a "sacrifice" in any true sense, because our health would improve in the process of reducing meat consumption. There are few totally vegetarian cultures in the world. However, Western culture is the only one that has made meat the centerpiece of its diet and has added the erroneous claim that we *need* it to survive.

While there are some who call upon us to examine moral and ethical reasons to decrease our meat consumption, I prefer to view the problem primarily as a health issue with global implications. That is the approach I am taking in this book. I want you to become aware of the benefits soy products offer you and your family and, at the same time, to think about the possibility that what is good for you is also good for our planet and the people who are currently competing for its resources. Ecological sense and health sense go hand in hand.

FAST FOOD SPREADS FAST

It is ironic that many east-Asian countries have been successfully penetrated by the U.S. fast-food industry. The fried chicken and hamburger franchises you are familiar with are becoming increasingly commonplace overseas, particularly in east-Asian urban centers. To compete with the influx of fast food chains, local merchants are establishing their own restaurants that feature food based on a Western diet. One major U.S. fast-food chain boasts *21,000 restaurants in over 100 countries.* If the hamburgers sold by this single company were placed in a chain, they would equal the distance of nineteen round trips from the earth to the moon! I am not criticizing these fast-food chains; after all, they are meeting an established consumer need. However, I forecast that they will start to produce vegetable protein dishes increasingly in the next decade or so.

United States fast-food leaders have long espoused a business philosophy characterized by the acronym QSCV, which stands for Quality, Service, Cleanliness, and Value. Unfortunately, "H for health" is not a part of this philosophy. Bowing to recent consumer concerns about health, the fat content of hamburgers has been reduced to a range of 17 to 20 percent of volume. This is small consolation when one considers that most of the fat in the meat is saturated fat, the type of fat that plays an important role in raising total blood cholesterol levels. High blood cholesterol (hypercholesterolemia) is a primary risk factor for coronary artery disease, the number one killer in our society.

While the picture I have painted sounds bleak indeed, and there clearly are global implications in the spread of fast food, there are promising signs. For example, one large franchise that features sandwiches is creating a competitive edge by stressing the low-fat content of its food compared with that served by other fast-food chains. Obviously, this chain is responding to concerns of educated consumers. It is possible that the fast-food industry will wake up and realize that they have much to learn about the benefits of soy protein. Perhaps one day soon we will see soy-burgers, soy milk, and soy yogurt offered as tasty and satisfying alternatives to a menu dominated by animal protein products.

That said, I invite you to read on and learn how soy has the potential to help you live a longer and healthier life. Although you might be reading this book because you are looking for help with specific health concerns, I recommend that you read the entire book in order to get more complete knowledge of the properties and uses of soy. By necessity, some of the information presented in this book is scientific. Although I have attempted to make the complex information accessible, it is impossible to provide a complete picture of the health benefits of soy without exploring in detail the chemical composition of soybeans and citing research that demonstrates its beneficial effects on many areas of human health.

Modern Medicine Engages Nutrition

Over the past two decades, medicine has reached a crossroads. Conventional ("allopathic") physicians are embroiled with practitioners of alternative (sometimes called "complementary" or "holistic") medicine, who often use nutritional or botanical interventions to treat and prevent disease. I reject this dichotomy in medicine and believe we should be preoccupied with what works rather than spend time fretting over the particular medical discipline from which a treatment emerges. Modern proponents of "integrated medicine" have done little to dispel this dichotomy, which will be resolved only by compromise and understanding. After all, it is health-care consumers, not health-care providers, who have the ultimate say in the therapy they receive, and many of them are seeking nutritional, natural alternatives to deal with their health problems.

The Research Is Convincing

There is no question that much of the evidence for the health benefits of soy foods emanate from population studies (epidemiology), where inconsistencies in the association between diseases and dietary habits or risk factors are common. Furthermore, the degree of importance of dietary constituents may vary, and one cannot be certain that multiple factors do not account for observed differences. For example, population studies show that soy diets are preventive against chronic degenerative diseases such as coronary artery disease and cancer. People who consume soy-based diets in Asian countries also have a lower incidence of breast or prostate cancer and heart disease, but their diets are also high in fiber and low in saturated fat, both of which may play a role in cancer prevention. I accept the limitations of epidemiological studies in proving a causal link between soy-based diets and disease prevention. However, one cannot ignore the ever-increasing number of basic science experiments and human clinical trials that show unequivocal health benefits for certain fractions of soybeans.

Speculations versus Facts

Throughout this book, I have attempted to separate speculation from scientific fact, but do not accept the arrogance of modern science that if something is not explicable in terms of current scientific theory then it is to be rejected. To set the stage for this book, I quote from the Preface of my first book, *Soya For Health*. That book was written primarily for health-care providers, but the interest in the book—which is found in many medical libraries—prompted me to write this book for the layperson.

> *I believe that the clear differences in disease profiles in the many Eastern versus Western communities are attributable to a major degree to the presence of soya in the diet. Of course, soya is not the panacea of health, but it operates as a major factor and determinant of the relative absence of certain killer diseases in several Asian societies.*
>
> *I am not alone in this belief, and several other authors have taken an opportunity to define some of health benefits of the soyabean. I have taken a large body of basic science and clinical research to formulate therapeutic concepts involving the use of soyabean fractions as nutriceuticals and general nutrients. It would be a shock to me if my clinical colleagues accepted all the therapeutic proposals that I have identified for soya, but I have the utmost confidence that physicians, health care professionals, and nutritionists will accept many of the suggestions.*

SOY: THE HEALTH FOOD OF THE NEXT MILLENNIUM

Strange things happen in science. I was both honored and anxious when I was invited to give my plenary lecture, "Soy: The Health Food of the Next Millennium," to the Korean Soybean Society during the International Symposium on Soymilk and Cow's milk in Seoul, Korea, in June, 1997. For a Westerner to talk about soy food for the next millennium in a country that has such a long history of the use of soy as a dietary staple is a daunting prospect.

I learned a great deal from this venture. According to the experts in Korea, the incorporation of traditional soy foods into East-Asian diets has peaked. These authorities believe that enhancing soy food consumption in Asian diets rests with the introduction of new forms of soy foods that have been largely developed in Western societies. Such formats include soy protein isolates, soy fiber products, and soybean oil products that have been developed by modern food technology research.

One of the leaders in the food technology field is Protein Technologies, Inc., a division of Ralston Purina, Inc. (whose parent company is Dow Chemical), headquartered in St. Louis. This company has contributed greatly to the research of development of health-giving fractions of soybeans that are used on a global basis. Protein Technologies, Inc., has been highly commended for its support of research that has shown the clear health benefits of soy foods, particularly their own high-quality protein isolates that are derived from soy.

A WORD ABOUT TERMS

Before moving on, it makes sense to discuss some terms you will encounter in this book. If you live in the United States, you are probably accustomed to hearing the words "soy" and "soybeans." These are the terms used for soy-based food products in the United States. However, *soya* is the more universal—and correct—term to use when discussing the variety of products derived from the soybean; it is the term I used in *Soya For Health*. However, because this book is published in the United States, I have used the more popular term, *soy*, throughout.

You will also encounter the term "fractionate" or "fraction." These terms refer to the ability to separate out particular components of soy and use and/or study them separately. Just as the term implies, these fractionates are part of the whole, but have potential value when separated from the whole.

The term "isolate," when used as a noun, refers to components that are removed from the whole, but retain their structural form. For example, soy protein isolates contain all the properties of the protein as found in the cultivated beans.

THE PROMISE OF SOY FOR THE NEXT MILLENNIUM

This book is designed to discuss the benefits of soy foods for preventing and treating many illnesses that plague Western societies. The causes of the various diseases and the role of soy in their potential prevention and treatment are presented as clearly as possible. Remember that the nutritional value of soy makes it an ideal source for use in dietary supplements and specific prevention and treatment programs. Adding soy foods to your diet can increase your general well-being. Table 1, below, provides a concise summary of some of the potential health benefits of soybeans.

TABLE 1
HYPOTHETICAL MECHANISMS FOR THE ROLE OF SOY DIETS
IN PROMOTION OF LONGEVITY

Condition	*Effect of Soy*
Premature death due to	
Heart disease	Promotes cardiovascular wellness
Hypertension and	
consequences	Lowers blood pressure
Cancer	Cancer preventive role
Renal failure	Potential renal benefits
Morbidity in old age due to	
Heart disease	Promotes cardiovascular wellness
Skeletal disorders	Certain soy foods prevent or treat osteoporosis
Cancer	Cancer preventive and therapeutic (?) role
Failing physiological functions	General good nutritional value

Soy Fractions for Health

Of all the components of soy-based products with a positive value for health, isoflavones lead the way. Isoflavones are phytoestrogens; that is, substances of plant origin that have effects similar to the female hormone estrogen. Isoflavones also have the capacity to modulate the effect of estrogens.

Genistein and another major isoflavone, daidzein, are the two major isoflavones that have sparked interest in the isoflavone components of soy foods. Well-defined results of epidemiological studies, in vitro laboratory experiments, tissue studies, animal experiments, and human studies support many of the claims of the anticancer effects of isoflavones have been reported in prostate, breast, colon, and skin cancer. Isoflavones have also been shown to prevent bone loss and decrease osteoporosis in animals and humans.

Soy Protein and Cholesterol

It has been recognized for approximately one hundred years that animal protein in the diet may promote atherosclerosis (a disease affecting the arterial walls) and that vegetable protein lowers cholesterol and, by inference, the risk of atheroma. Atheroma is the build up of fatty deposits on the lining of the arteries that can then cause atherosclerosis. Cholesterol-lowering drugs have come into increasing use, but they may be unnecessary in many cases because soy protein in the diet is effective for treating most types of hypercholesterolemia (high levels of cholesterol in the blood).

Recently, James Anderson, M.D., has presented an excellent statistical analysis of reports of clinical studies that show substantial reductions of blood cholesterol by using soy protein supplements or by switching to soy protein as the primary source of protein in the diet. It should be noted that the levels of these reductions in blood cholesterol and other fat compounds in the blood are similar to those achieved with maintenance doses of synthetic drugs. However, the reductions of blood lipids brought on by the synthetic drugs come at a price, both in terms of monetary cost and the suffering brought on by side effects. Since this is true, it is more than a little bewildering that health-care professionals or patients would use them without first trying the soy protein supplement. Soy has a demonstrable ability to lower blood lipids, and I consider it to be a first-line option in treating high cholesterol.

Soy and Osteoporosis

Landmark studies have been performed on the relationship between animal protein-rich diets and calcium metabolism, especially in relationship to the formation of kidney stones. In these studies, individuals consumed diets containing varying amounts of calcium and protein of either plant or animal origin. Subjects were divided into three groups. One ate protein derived from meat or cheese; a second consumed protein from cheese, eggs, soy milk, or texturized vegetable protein; and the third consumed protein from soy products only. Those who consumed animal protein lost about 50 percent more calcium in their urine than those who ate soy protein alone.

The reasons that soy protein isolates may protect against calcium loss from the body are not entirely clear, but are probably related to their amino acid content. Soy protein tends to be low in sulfur-containing amino acids, and sulfate compounds may inhibit the reabsorption of calcium by the kidneys, thereby promoting hypercalciuria (excessive calcium loss through the urine). The mechanisms of nutrient-related causes of calcium loss remain poorly understood, and when finally known, are likely to be more complex than hitherto discussed. For example, protein of animal origin is known to contain relatively high levels of phosphorus or phosphates, which may result in loss of calcium in the stool. However, phosphorus may assist in the conservation of calcium in the kidneys. These findings illustrate some of the complexities of the factors that operate in maintaining stable levels of calcium in the body.

The increased understanding of the role of isoflavones contained within soy protein isolates has resulted in new insight into the beneficial effects of soy protein on skeletal health. An isoflavone-related compound, ipriflavone, has been found to be effective in reducing bone loss in animals and humans with osteoporosis. When ipriflavone is metabolized it converts, in part, to form the isoflavone daidzein, a component of certain soy protein isolates.

Osteoarthritis is often associated with osteoporosis, and evidence has emerged that it is amenable to therapy with compounds that have an antiangiogenic effect, meaning that they interfere with blood vessel growth. Angiogenesis—that is, new blood vessel growth—is associated with osteoarthritis, cancer, and other chronic disorders, and this has led to a proposal that dietary supplements with antiangiogenic effects may be useful in the treatment of these diseases. Although it is notable that isoflavones, especially genistein, contained within soy protein isolates, are antiangiogenic, the specific role of isoflavones in preventing or treating diseases associated with unwanted new blood vessel growth (angiogenesis) still needs further clarification.

Soy Protein and Kidney Function

Evidence has accumulated showing that vegetable-based protein, particularly soy protein, is much more efficiently handled by the kidneys than animal protein. Beneficial effects of soy diets on high blood cholesterol in patients with kidney impairment due to nephrotic syndrome have been reported. Nephrotic syndrome is a kidney disease that results in protein loss in the urine with variable degrees of water retention (edema), high blood pressure (hypertension), and high levels of fats in the blood (blood lipids). It has been found that switching from a predominately animal protein source to a vegetarian (soy) source of protein results in a substantial decrease in both blood cholesterol and protein loss from the kidneys in individuals with this and other types of kidney failure.

Studies of kidney, metabolic, and hormonal responses to animal and vegetable protein diets show that considerable benefits may result from vegetable protein-based diets. It has been found that animal protein causes a glomerular filtration rate (the filtering mechanism of the kidneys) that is about one-fifth higher than that caused by soy protein. These studies imply that instead of making drastic reductions in protein intake in patients with kidney failure, it may be possible to switch the protein source in the diet from animal to soy-based protein. Since kidney function decreases with age, soy protein is an attractive option as a source of protein in the diets of the elderly.

Prostatic Disease and Soy

Several studies have drawn attention to the lower incidence of prostatic disease in Japanese men compared with Western men. The difference is particularly clear in older men. The difference in prevalence of prostatic disease has been ascribed in part to the high intake of soy foods in the Japanese diet. The isoflavone content of soy (genistein and daidzein) has been shown to directly affect testosterone metabolism and to help reduce the formation of toxic types of testosterone. The benefits of soy-based diets in the promotion of prostatic health have led to the recommendation that men at risk of prostate problems take soy daily in their diet.

There is a great deal more research to be done in this area. In the meantime alternative and contemporary health-care practitioners have taken the lead in the use of soy to prevent and treat prostatic disease. A notable example is the Michael B. Schachter Prostaplan, which contains the soy-based drink Prostagen.

Soy and Hypertension

Japanese investigators have shed some light on the antihypertensive effects of soybean diets. Studies have shown that fermented soy foods, such as natto and miso, may contain antihypertensive peptides that may interfere with blood pressure regulation. (Peptides are chains of amino acids that occur in a specific sequence.) Further studies are underway to confirm these findings, but it appears that these peptides may interfere with angiotensin-converting enzyme, an enzyme that promotes the production of angiotensin, which, in turn, causes elevated blood pressure. It is important to realize that inhibitors of angiotensin-converting enzymes are among the most widely used synthetic pharmaceuticals in standard medical practice for the control of hypertension. It would appear that nature has already provided the key to control hypertension in the form of soy.

Estrogenic Effects of Soy

Discussed in detail in Chapter 3, soy isoflavones are capable of binding an estrogen receptor in the body. This activity appears to be related to a potential benefit of soy in preventing breast cancer or even in the treatment of the disease. Controlled studies are underway to examine the benefits of soy diets or supplements in breast cancer therapy.

Another very interesting application of the estrogenic effect of soy isoflavones is the potential management of menopausal symptoms. It has been noted that Japanese women, who often consume large amounts of soy, may have a much lower prevalence of menopausal symptoms than Western women. This is believed to be related to the biological effects of isoflavones as estrogens. The Sloan-Kettering Cancer Center and Iowa State University, as well as other major institutions, are engaged in research of soy isoflavones in the potential control of menopausal symptoms.

Information Sources

Many health benefits of soybeans have been recognized in basic science and clinical literature. Soybeans are an ever-increasing source of dietary supplements that will become available as over-the-counter products. Further information on sources of dietary supplements that can be derived from soy are available by writing to: The Soy Information Department, Biotherapies, Inc., 9 Commerce Road, Fairfield, New Jersey 07004, or by fax only at 973/276-0639.

The following chapter discusses some of the important components of soy and the variety of ways soy can be consumed.

CHAPTER 2

"What Makes Soybeans So Special?"

Soy is usually discussed as a single entity—as a particular food—but soy is consumed in numerous forms, each of which has its own nutrient profile. For example, dry-roasted soybeans are often consumed as a snack food and are a good source of nutrients and fiber. However, liquid soy products, such as soy milk, contain only small amounts of soluble fiber.

Soy oil is sometimes hydrogenated during processing so that it contains more saturated fatty acids than the unprocessed form of the oil. It is unfortunate that much of the soybean oil used in the North American diet is the unhealthy hydrogenated type. I do not believe that hydrogenated plant oils are healthy. They may contain dangerous types of trans-fatty acids. So the idea that margarine, which is really hydrogenated vegetable oil, is healthy requires reappraisal.

As you will see, soy is a versatile food, but we can reap its great benefits only by knowing the best ways to use it. Boiled soybeans and tofu are sources of calcium, but the calcium content of soy milk varies greatly, depending on the brand one purchases. Certain components, or "fractions," of soybeans, such as isoflavones (discussed below and in detail in Chapter 3), have clear "medicinal" benefits. In order to achieve these benefits, they need to be given in predictable amounts on a regular basis. For this reason, it makes good sense to consider using dietary supplements for isoflavones and other soy fractions.

When we look at the overall composition of soybeans, we can see that their potential to prevent and treat disease is significant. We have also reached a critical juncture in the research, a point where past supposition and speculation have been transformed into concrete evidence that we can use to improve our health and help prevent various conditions and diseases.

Following is a brief summary of some of the beneficial nutritional components of soybeans. Additional information is found in relevant sections of this book, which discuss specific health concerns and the application of soy.

Fiber: Fiber is an all-inclusive term used for the substances in plant foods that remain virtually unchanged as they travel through the digestive tract. Some fiber that is found in many vegetables and in wheat is firm and often described as crunchy, or insoluble. The fiber found in oats is described as soluble, or sticky. Soybeans contain both soluble and insoluble types of fiber. The fact that soybeans contain both insoluble and soluble fibers means that soy can help regulate gastrointestinal function and reduce cholesterol levels.

Vitamins and Minerals: Soybeans are packed with important nutrients, including calcium, magnesium, and many B-complex vitamins. Eat a half-cup of boiled soybeans, and you have consumed almost half (about 44 percent) the Recommended Daily Allowance (RDA) of iron. You will also receive a significant amount of calcium, magnesium, and zinc. Thiamine, niacin, riboflavin, and vitamin B_6 are also present in amounts significant enough to consider soybeans a good source of these B-complex vitamins. Mature soybeans are not a source of vitamin C, but soybean sprouts are.

Soy isoflavones also function as antioxidants. In this role they neutralize the effects of free radicals, which have the ability to damage cells and impair immunity. Antioxidants are believed to have a significant role in preventing cancer or retarding its growth. The indications that soy contains many valuable anticancer substances are so strong that it has become the subject of many cancer prevention studies.

Flavonoids: This group of chemicals is largely responsible for the yellow, red, or deep blue color in fruits and flowers. *Bio*flavonoids are found in citrus fruits, and interest in them increased when 1937 Nobel Laureate of Medicine/Physiology Albert Szent-Györgyi demonstrated that the bioflavonoids in citrus fruits, act like a vitamin in the body. Bioflavonoids are vitamin C helpers, among other things. Szent-Györgyi's research led to further investigation, and flavonoids have been discovered in numerous foods, including soybeans. They are thought to have significant anti-cancer properties and act to inhibit enzymes that stimulate cancer growth in its early stages.

Isoflavones: Isoflavones hold the key to understanding the versatile and powerful health benefits of soy. These compounds are polyphenols (cancer-fighting compounds), which are related to one of the fifteen classes of flavonoids, and they are phytoalexins, chemicals a plant produces to protect itself under stressful conditions. Isoflavones are particularly important in our discussion of cancer because they are phytoestrogens, meaning that they have a structure that mimics the hormone estrogen, and they are involved in balancing estrogen's effects in the body. Again, the prefix *phyto* indicates that these estrogens occur in plants. The story is more complex, however, because it appears that in some circumstances, isoflavones actually negate harmful effects of estrogen (they act as antiestrogens) and may therefore play a role in preventing certain types of breast cancer—and other cancers as well. Soy is the single most important source of phytoestrogens, making it potentially one of the premier foods involved in preventing some forms of cancer. Genistein and daidzein are two important phytoestrogens found in soybeans. The ability of soy isoflavones to prevent and treat cancer of the breast and prostate is currently being investigated in several multimillion-dollar research projects.

Miscellaneous Polyphenols: These compounds are also anticancer chemicals that are abundant in soybeans and a few other plants. They act as a form of "chemical garbage collectors" as they go about neutralizing cancer causing agents in the body. It is believed that these substances interfere with other chemicals that promote tumor growth. Therefore, they play a valuable role in suppressing the growth of cancerous cells in the body.

Terpenes, Saponins, and Phytosterols: Often found in plant oils and resins, these compounds interrupt cancer cell formation, thereby helping to negate the harmful effects of cancer-causing substances. Saponins have antioxidant properties, and further investigation is needed to determine their exact role in preventing cancer; specifically, solid tumors such as colon cancer. Saponins may also play a part in controlling cholesterol levels by interfering with its absorption from the gastrointestinal tract.

Found only in plants, phytosterols resemble cholesterol in their chemical structure, but these chemicals may help prevent heart disease rather than contribute to it. Phytosterols are not absorbed into the body from the intestines; instead, they move to the colon, where they may exert a potential role in protecting against colon cancer.

Phytates: Phytates contain a very important mineral, phosphorus. They are sometimes considered to be potentially harmful in that they bind with other minerals, such as iron, and prevent their absorption in the intestines. However, the antinutrient characteristic of phytates that was once thought to be harmful may instead be what gives phytate its ability to protect against colon cancer. When phytate binds with iron, free radical formation is inhibited. In this situation, phytate is acting as an antioxidant substance. So, rather than being detrimental to health because it inhibits iron absorption, phytate may act to keep iron at a safe level in the body. Some experiments suggest that phytates may also enhance the immune system and have a role controlling cell growth.

HOW DO WE CONSUME THIS "WONDER" FOOD?

Tofu, tempeh, soy milk, soy cheese, and miso are only a few of the foods available derived from soy beans. The versatility of this plant means that it offers something for everyone. Below is a list of some of the soy products you will find in typical natural food markets or, quite often nowadays, in conventional grocery stores.

Dried soybeans: Soybeans are a member of the legume family, and can be used much like other leguminous dried beans. They can be baked or boiled alone or with a mixture of beans and vegetables and also added to soup and casseroles. Cooked whole, soybeans retain their fiber content.

Fresh soybeans: Although not yet popular in the West, immature soybeans can be cooked in the pod, and then removed and served as a vegetable or as a snack. Some Asian restaurants are now featuring steamed fresh soybeans, indicating that this dish may be rising in popularity. The pod alone is sometimes used in stir fry dishes. It is not easy to find fresh soybeans, even in health food markets, but this is likely to change as soy becomes a larger part of our dietary landscape.

Soy nuts: These are either dry-roasted or deep-fried, and are eaten as a snack food. While an excellent source of protein and isoflavones, this snack food is high in salt and fat that has been denatured (broken down and changed) by heat. Soy nuts should be eaten sparingly, much the way we consume peanuts or sesame seeds.

Soy sprouts: Sprouted soy beans are high in vitamin C, as are other sprouted seeds. Soybean sprouts can be used raw on salads or cooked in stir-fry dishes. As sprouts of all kinds are more readily available, soy sprouts also appear. Soybeans can be sprouted at home quite easily, in a manner similar to alfalfa seeds or mung beans.

Tofu: Tofu is produced by adding a curdling agent to soy milk, thereby separating the substance into curds and a form of whey. The curds are then put into molds and left to stand; within a few hours, the curds are formed into firm blocks. Much of the tofu we see in today's supermarkets is packaged in water to keep it fresh, which is the way it has been stored for centuries.

One of the most popular soy products, tofu comes in many varieties and is used in multiple ways. Also known as bean curd, tofu has been around for a long time—it was probably first produced about 2,000 years ago. One Chinese legend tells us that tofu was invented by a government official, who, because he refused to take bribes, was so poor that he experimented with soybeans and came up with tofu, a dish he could afford on his modest salary. Another story credits a Chinese alchemist for inventing, or perhaps we should say, discovering, the potential of using a by-product of soy milk, which was named "tofu." Buddhist monks from China introduced tofu to Japan, where it became a food considered so important—and sacred—that it is sometimes referred to as *o-tofu*, the prefix indicating the designation of "honorable."

Tofu absorbs other flavors, which is why, in our culture anyway, it is often used as a substitute for meat and dairy products. Many excellent cookbooks are available that describe how to use tofu as a substitute for cheese in lasagna, for example, or even as a substitute for cream cheese in cheesecake. Tofu is also a favorite protein source for stir-fry dishes and as an addition to miso soup. Certain types of tofu are increasingly popular as frozen desserts, which represent more healthful alternatives to ice cream.

Tofu is a low-fat, low-sodium, high-protein food. It is a plant food that does not contain cholesterol, and can be an excellent source of isoflavones if consumed in large enough quantities (*e.g.*, greater than eight ounces per day). Only a few years ago, tofu was used as an example of the kind of food "health nuts" consumed, but today it has made its way into mainstream markets. In fact, about 75 percent of the tofu consumed in the U.S. is purchased in conventional supermarkets.

The best source of information on the history of the development, manufacture, and application of tofu is found in *The Book of Tofu*, by William Shurtleff and his wife, Akiko Aoyagi Shurtleff.

Tempeh: Tempeh is a fermented product made from soybeans that have been soaked and cooked to soften them. Like sourdough bread, tempeh requires a starter substance, which is added to the cooked beans. This mixture is left for twenty-four hours, and the result is a firm, textured product with a somewhat nutty flavor and a texture similar to a chewy mushroom. Because tempeh is firm and it can be formed into a patty, it is often used as a substitute for animal products.

This soy product is especially popular in Indonesia and is considered a national specialty. It has the necessary characteristics of a dietary staple in that is high in protein and fiber and is rich in other nutrients. It also has the advantage of containing vitamin B_{12}, which is a by-product of the fermentation process.

A striking breakthrough in the production of soy for dietary supplementation has been made by BioFoods, Inc., of Wayne, New Jersey. This company uses fermentation processes to produce a product that contains isoflavones in a format that is easy for the body to absorb.

Soy milk: Soy milk is made by adding water to full-fat soy flour or by soaking ground soybeans in water and turning the mixture into a smooth liquid. It is sometimes patronizingly described as an "adequate substitute" for dairy products, without mentioning any of the negative features of dairy, such as its saturated fat and cholesterol content. In fact, **I believe that there is no reason to consume dairy products preferentially when we have soy milk available as a healthful substitute**. While it does not taste exactly like cow's milk, the taste is close enough that most people quickly adjust to it. Soy milk can be purchased in flavored varieties, such as an added nutty taste, or with favorites of the Western palate—vanilla, chocolate, and apple. Using soy milk is a simple way to add soy products to your diet.

Miso: This is another fermented soy product, made by mixing softened soybeans, water, and salt into a paste. The starter substance is made from a grain such as rice or barley; fungal organisms, notably aspergillus oryzae, are also used in the process. Traditionally, the mixture is aged in cedar vats. It is used to flavor soup, salad dressings, and other dishes. Miso is a staple food in Japanese cooking, and a bowl of miso soup is often part of a traditional Japanese breakfast.

Rich in protein and isoflavones, miso is often loaded with salt and should be incorporated into the diet in moderation. It is not an appropriate food for people on salt-restricted diets. The occurrence of stroke due to hemorrhage into the brain and gastric cancer are more common among Japanese people than in people from many other nations. High salt intake in the diet may be the culprit.

Soy concentrates: When soy protein is isolated (referred to as soy protein isolate), it can be consumed in powdered form and used in many products, from infant formula to meal replacement preparations used in weight-loss programs. Some athletes regularly use this protein powder while they are training. If you use nondairy creamer, it is likely that you have consumed soy protein isolate because it is used often as a replacement for milk. The powdered form is also used as a meat extender or as an additive in certain prepared foods.

Soy flour: Soy flour is either derived from finely ground soybeans, or produced as a by-product of soy food and soy milk manufacturing. In its common form it is about 50 percent protein, and it is used extensively in some varieties of commercial baked goods. More recently it has become available to consumers for home baking. Since soy does not contain gluten, it is not used for baking that requires yeast and cannot be used as the primary flour in raised breads. It is sold in both full-fat and defatted forms.

Texturized soy protein (TSP): Texturized soy protein can be transformed into a meat substitute, making sausage, hamburger, and chili that has the desirable balance of omega-3 and omega-6 essential fatty acids that the beef lacks. Adding soy protein to ground beef or sausage, in addition to giving some fatty acid benefits, decreases the calorie density of the meat, making it more acceptable in a weight-loss program, not to mention making the meat more tender and juicy. Texturized soy protein is high in protein and is a good source of isoflavones and certain minerals, including calcium. Soy protein and fiber also can be used to make a delicious soy-flake cereal.

Some commercially produced meat substitutes using soy contain sodium, dyes, and other additives. *Read the labels care-*

fully. VitaPro, located in Montreal, Canada, and BioFoods, located in Wayne, New Jersey, are two leaders in the development of these products.

Soybean Oil: Soy oil has found a home in many commercial food products, from salad dressing to baked goods. Surprisingly, soybean oil is one of the most common sources of calories in Western diets. While it is beneficial in many ways, it should not be overconsumed because it can add unwanted calories in the form of fat to your diet. As a plant food, soy is low in saturated fat (about 15 percent). Of the polyunsaturated fat in soy oil, a good portion is linoleic acid of the omega-6 type, a fatty acid we need in significant amounts. In addition, soy oil contains an important and beneficial fatty acid, linolenic acid, an omega-3 fatty acid precursor. Omega-3 fatty acids are found primarily in fish oils in their free form. Linolenic acid is a precursor of DHA (docosahexaenoic acid) and EPA (eicosapentaenoic acid), which have important functions in maintaining memory and brain development as well as fighting inflammation in the body. Omega-3 fatty acids are believed to be helpful in preventing heart disease and several other chronic degenerative diseases. Soy oil is an important source of omega-3 fatty acids for vegetarians and others who do not consume fish.

Soy oil is found in so many food products that it would be difficult to find many commercially prepared baked goods that do not contain at least some soy oil. Margarines and solid shortenings contain soy oil, as do many processed meat products. This does not mean that the products are any more healthful, however. When soy oil is used commercially it is usually partially hydrogenated, meaning that it is no longer polyunsaturated and the essential fatty acid content is reduced. In addition, hydrogenation produces types of fatty acids, called trans-fatty acids, that can even raise blood cholesterol levels and precipitate adverse cardiovascular events. It is ironic that with all the health benefits that soybeans offer, the typical U.S. diet features large amounts of processed soy oil, perhaps the least nutritionally important component of this special legume. Of course, this is explained by the fact that the U.S. is an important producer of soybeans and soybean oil is relatively inexpensive, not to mention versatile.

Soy sauce: Virtually everyone has consumed soy sauce, and it is no doubt one of the most popular seasonings on the planet. It is a fermented product made from soybeans and wheat, with aspergillus mold spores added. It comes in many varieties, from salty and dense to slightly sweet and light. Unfortunately, a lot of soy sauce is a major source of unwanted salt in the diet. There are imitation soy sauces on the market, so we must read labels carefully if we want the highest quality product. Tamari is similar to soy sauce and is usually sold in health food markets. Low-sodium soy sauce and tamari are also available.

READ THE LABELS

The foods listed above are the most common soy foods you are likely to encounter. A stroll through a progressive type of food market is instructive in learning just how versatile soybeans are. While you will see many products, from many varieties of miso and tofu to several different brands of soy milk and soy flour, you will also see soy frozen desserts and even cinnamon rolls made with tofu. However, a food made with soy is not healthful if its ingredients also include large quantities of sugar and fat, and commercial products don't become "natural" foods just because they are made with soy oil. So, be a careful label reader, no matter where you shop.

SOY AS A "NUTRICEUTICAL," OR DIETARY SUPPLEMENT

Although the term nutriceutical is relatively new, the concept is not. For example, for many years iodine was added to salt to prevent goiter. As a result, goiter, enlargement of the thyroid gland due to iodine deficiency, has been virtually eliminated as a medical condition. More recently folic acid has been added to food to prevent birth defects of the spinal cord and brain stem.

An important example of a soy nutriceutical are the soy isoflavones. These soy fractions are phytoestrogens, and have great potential for use in estrogen replacement therapy for menopausal women. Many brands of isoflavone supplements are available. Phyto-Est, from Biotherapies of Fairfield, New Jersey, and Soynatto from BioFoods of Wayne, New Jersey, are two that are produced to careful standards.

It is important to remember that the use of soy isoflavones as "hormonal" therapy has not been approved by the FDA. The Dietary and Health Education Act of 1994 imposes very strict guidelines that do not permit dietary supplements—nutriceuticals—to be sold for use in preventing or treating any disease. On the other hand, in most cases, consumers can buy and use these products to prevent and treat medical disorders. This is a modern contention in health care.

DRUGS FAIL AND NUTRITION MAY BE THE ANSWER!

Let's Digress

Americans spend more than sixty billion dollars per year on prescription medications. This could be considered a major public investment in health, yet these dollars have not had a pervasive impact on the many causes of premature death and disability. In fact, some prescription and over-the-counter medications have become the focus of public health concerns. For example, non-steroidal anti-inflammatory drugs (NSAIDs), such as aspirin, ibuprofen, naproxen, and so forth, account for a significant amount of kidney and liver impairment in the elderly population. In several research studies, my colleagues and I have shown that these medications are also one of the most frequent causes of life-threatening bleeding from the stomach and bowel. These drugs are misused and sometimes misprescribed. There are alternatives to NSAIDs

Cardiovascular disease remains the number one killer in Western society. As the link between high blood cholesterol and heart disease is increasingly recognized, hundreds of thousands of people are given prescriptions for synthetic drugs that lower fats in the blood. These drugs have a good record for effectiveness, yet they are often offered without seriously considering the many dietary and lifestyle changes that can reduce blood cholesterol. Dietary and lifestyle changes that patients institute themselves are without side effects, and have the potential to enhance over-all health and well-being, rather than treat just one condition or disease. As you will see in Chapter 4, soy protein lowers blood cholesterol very efficiently, and, as a low-cost, widely available, and safe alternative to drug therapy, it has no equal.

While I cannot promote the use of soy to treat or prevent AIDS, plant saponins (and other compounds) in soy are known to interfere with the proliferation of the AIDS virus. Soy also provides a good dietary base for individuals with AIDS. Its ver-satility means that it can be engineered to provide excellent sup-plementary food and nutrients for the individual with nutritional problems due to immunodeficiency.

If humankind is to progress in the areas of disease preven-tion and treatment, then we must begin to explore natural resources that have been used for thousands of years. Bringing modern scientific methods to these resources may show us the way to save ourselves untold suffering. I hope my speculation prompts more research into remedies of natural origin.

CHAPTER 3

The Ingenious Soy Isoflavones

Soy isoflavones are a unique group of phytoestrogens: that is, estrogens of plant origin. This chapter will show you how they can be either proestrogenic or antiestrogenic, depending on the estrogen balance present in the body of the person ingesting them. Thus, we can begin to think of soy isoflavones not only as estrogens but as compounds that modulate—or balance—estrogenic effects in the body. Another way to say this is that they are "adaptogens," substances that help restore balance to the human body.

There is no question that estrogen can be a woman's best friend. Menstruation and fertility are dependent on the presence of estrogen, and without this hormone, the female sex characteristics do not develop. At times, however, estrogen can be a woman's worst enemy. Estrogen is implicated in a variety of women's health complaints, such as premenstrual syndrome (PMS), some symptoms of the menopause, and mastalgia (breast pain). It also plays a role in the development of certain types of breast cancer and other types of estrogen-dependent cancers.

The negative side of estrogen does not affect women exclusively. Under some circumstances, estrogen appears to "facilitate" the development of benign prostate enlargement.

THE ORIGIN OF PSEUDOESTROGENS

The modern human diet contains an array of synthetic and natural compounds that can mimic estrogen and its related forms. In addition, several man-made estrogens have crept into the human diet in a variety of ways. Most people do not realize or even suspect that these exist. For example, many herbicides and pesticides used routinely in the agricultural industry have estrogenic activity, and food processing does not easily remove these chemicals. Unfortunately, synthetic estrogens are also introduced from plastics and packaging materials. Added to those sources is the deliberate use of synthetic estrogens in the contraceptive pill, used by millions of women of reproductive age, and hormone replacement therapy (HRT), given to millions of women at the time of menopause.

The estrogen-like hormones used to promote growth that are added to domestic animal and poultry feeds are of great concern. These hormones are used to enhance meat production; that is, they produce animals that are ready for consumption in as little time as possible. Some of us may choke on a forkful of turkey or chicken raised with these hormones if we paused to assess the possible effects that these chemical agents have on our bodies.

Mycotoxins are compounds produced by various species of a particular type of mold. These mycotoxins are estrogenic in their action, and they commonly infect cereal products. This represents another "hidden" source of estrogen that we consume widely in our diet.

A Closer Look

Practically all commercial fruits and vegetables have traces of pesticides, and animal products such as milk, dairy foods, and fish contain these agents to varying degrees. It goes without saying that all fruits and vegetables should be washed before eating. It is unfortunate that some soybean crops are contaminated with pesticides, too, although food processing eliminates many of these contaminants. However, soy products made from organically grown soybeans are available and are preferred when you have a choice. Unfortunately, there have been concerns raised about soybeans coming from some countries in Eastern Asia that are certified as organic but have been found to contain undesirable amounts of herbicides and pesticides. This situation has been used as a powerful argument for genetic engineering of soybeans to produce varieties that are resistant to infection and infestation.

Naturally occurring estrogens in foods—those that are not synthetic contaminants—can be classified into several different categories. Major categories of botanical estrogens are isoflavones (found in soy), lignins (from plant fibers) coumestans (found mainly in clover and alfalfa, but also present in germinated soybeans and other legumes), and resorcylic acid lactones (zearalone and related compounds), which are mycotoxins. Obviously, the whole story of pseudoestrogens is quite complex, and to fully understand it, one needs a knowledge of chemistry and physiology. However, three soy isoflavones—daidzein, genistein, and glycetin—are considered the most important and have attracted wide interest because of their potential health benefits. One thing is clear: these isoflavones offer versatile health benefits, and their value extends to a great many areas of human health.

GROUNDBREAKING RESEARCH EXPLAINS THE ACTION OF ESTROGENS AND SOY ISOFLAVONES

In 1997, peer-reviewed medical literature was alive with scientific reports of new discoveries about the way estrogens act in the human body. It is now recognized that there are at least two types of estrogen receptors in the cells, which have been termed alpha and beta receptors. The "classic" estrogen receptor was known to reside in the nucleus of the cells, but there is evidence that there are receptors in the cell sap (cytoplasm) of cells that also respond to the cellular messages given by estrogenic compounds.

Over the past seven years, scientist Mark Messina has reviewed a great deal of information on the health benefits of soy. In his presentation entitled "The Renaissance of Soy" at the 1997 National Nutritional Foods Association (NNFA) Annual Meeting in Las Vegas, Dr. Messina reported that in 1985, a computer search of the literature revealed only a handful of papers on isoflavones; in the past three years, however, more than one thousand papers have appeared on the effects of soy isoflavones, especially in relationship to their anti-cancer effects.

Dr. Messina also pointed to the rapid growth of interest in the use of soy isflavones in dietary supplement format. About forty companies produce isoflavone supplements alone or in combination with other putative phytochemicals for a variety of alleged health benefits.

Although isoflavones are weak estrogens and estrogen itself has been implicated as a cause of cancer, the question remains: How do soy isoflavones (phytoestrogens) prevent cancer? Dr. Messina supports the widely accepted theory that isoflavones can function in some circumstances as an antiestrogen. The antiestrogenic potential of isoflavones includes their ability to compete with or bind estrogen receptors, thereby preventing the action of the body's own estrogens. Other issues are important, such as increasing the level of sex binding globulin in the blood, which makes less free estrogen available to have an estrogenic effect.

The whole issue of how isoflavones exert an anticancer effect remains unclear or is disputed. Dr. David Zava, in a lecture given at the NNFA 1997 meeting, highlighted his work that showed unequivocally that genistein has anticancer effects that are unrelated to its ability to interfere with the actions of estrogen. Thus, the anticancer effects of soy isoflavones involve mechanisms other than hormonal effects in the body.

Mark Messina has discussed some of the evidence that soy isoflavones are protective against breast cancer, and he believes that soy isoflavones may have a predominantly estrogenic effect on the breast. Unlike many other authorities, Dr. Messina has questioned—in part—the protective role of soy isoflavones against breast cancer occurring in adults, but he creates a strong argument for their chemoprotective effects against cancer.

Some very interesting data have emerged in animal experiments that show that soy administered early in life may protect against breast cancer later in life. When groups of animals receive genistein early in life for three days and are then given a breast cancer carcinogen (an agent that promotes breast cancer), the occurrence of breast cancer is diminished one-hundred-fold among the animals given genistein early in life. I believe that soy isoflavones exert protection against breast cancer when administered to both adults and children, and they may have a role in the treatment of certain types of breast cancer.

ESTROGEN RECEPTORS: CAUSE FOR CONFUSION

The body's own estrogens, most notably estradiol, bind to certain locations in cells in the body where estrogen exerts an effect. Estrogen has a major role as a sex hormone but it is also trophic, which means that it stimulates growth or causes cells to divide or proliferate. Estrogen binds to receptors, which then give messages through chemical reactions for cells to work in a certain way. The cells comprise target tissues like uterine, breast, and bone tissues. The receptors for estrogen in these target tissues are triggered in the presence of estrogen (or isoflavones). Therefore, estrogen has many different effects throughout the body, and its effect on one tissue may not be the same as on another. Thus, estrogen-like molecules—soy isoflavones, for example—and estrogen may act through the same estrogen receptors, but they may display very different activities in different cells. This is why isoflavones can act like estrogens at one time, with a proestrogenic effect, or act at another time against the action of estrogens in an antiestrogenic effect.

IS SOY AN ALTERNATIVE FOR ESTRO-GEN REPLACEMENT THERAPY?

Dr. Gregory Burke, vice chairman of the Department of Public Health Science at Bowman Gray School of Medicine of Wake Forest University in North Carolina, has asked this question and answered it with a qualified "yes." Estrogen replacement therapy (ERT) is the most commonly filled prescription in community pharmacies in North America. To take or not to take ERT is a decision made by forty million mature women in the United States. Conventional ERT is taken by only 15 to 20 percent of menopausal women, and it is estimated that large numbers of women who received prescriptions for ERT never even fill the prescription because they fear the consequences of this therapy. As the population of the U.S. and other Western societies live longer, the issue of ERT in menopausal women becomes even bigger.

The rationale for ERT with conventional preparations is sound, but standard ERT carries a risk of the promotion of breast cancer, uterine cancer, and vascular thrombosis (blood clot). ERT is often effective at reducing menopausal symptoms, preventing osteoporosis, preventing coronary artery disease, benefiting urinary function, and perhaps preventing Alzheimer's disease. However, standard ERT is not safe, and isoflavones from soy are known to reduce menopausal symptoms, prevent and perhaps treat osteoporosis, prevent coronary artery disease, exert an antithrombolic effect (in contrast to the thrombolic effects of estrogens) and act as a powerful antioxidant. In contrast to standard ERT, soy isoflavones are safe and natural.

WHERE TO GET YOUR SOY ISOFLAVONES

The health benefits of isoflavones are dependent on continuous intake of soy foods in the diet. However, problems arise both in the relatively low *consistent* consumption of soy foods among

Westerners and the great variability of the isoflavone ⟨
soy foods.

Food processing techniques that use solvents (*e.g.*, aqueous
alcoholic solutions) may remove isoflavones from soy foods,
thereby making the total isoflavone content unpredictable. This
adds, of course, to the fundamental question about the willingness and ability among Westerners to add sufficient soy foods to
their diet to ingest the optimal amount of isoflavones. For the
most part, most Westerners find it unacceptable to eat eight to
ten ounces (more than one half pound) of tofu per day, for example, in order to ingest 50 to 80 mg of isoflavones per day.

From the mid part of 1996 to date, it has been impossible to
find a women's magazine that has not carried a story on the health
benefits of soy foods, especially in relationship to their potential
for menopausal well-being and the management of premenstrual
syndrome (PMS). Isoflavones are the active ingredient in soy that
effectively suppresses menopausal symptoms and promotes cardiovascular and bone health in the mature female. Therefore, the
idea that tofu is the answer requires some reappraisal.

Not all tofu contains significant quantitities of isoflavones,
and tofu is a traditional soy dish that does not have a general
appeal to the Western palate. As a result, something very unfortunate has happened. Menopausal women have taken a couple of
spoons of tofu for a week or two and then rejected the dietary
intervention because they have not achieved the desired effect.
But not all tofu is created equal, and consumers need ways to
obtain predictable amounts of isoflavones that will produce the
optimal health outcome. This reasoning supports the use of
dietary supplements made from fractions of soy for predictable
effects.

Soy milk represents a practical alternative to dairy milk and
is relatively easy to add to the diet. The best prepared products
contain about 12 mg of total isoflavones per 100 ml, and 400 ml
of soy milk per day is a very good health drink for mature men and
women. However, some forms of soy milk contain only small
amounts of isoflavones.

Concerns about the practical availability of soy isoflavones in the diet have led innovative dietary supplement manufacturers to formulate products that are convenient to take and also offer predictable isoflavone content. The first such product to be marketed was Phyto-Est, which contains a soy isoflavone concentrate of soy protein formulated in capsules. Three capsules of Phyto-Est, taken each day, provide about 50 to 60 mg of total isoflavones (genistein, daidzein, and the minor isoflavone, glycetein). At last count, there were more than fifty brands of isoflavone-containing dietary supplements on the market, and many contain the wrong amount of isoflavones to acheive the desired health benefits for menopause.

Other convenient soy isoflavone supplements come in the form of soy protein isolate powders. Genista is an example of such a product. Powdered, miscible (able to be mixed) beverages based on soy protein and isoflavone concentrates that can be combined with water or milk are also available. Prostagen and FemSoy are two such products. FemSoy, a drink mix powder, is increasingly used by women seeking relief from menopausal symptoms or problems associated with premenstrual syndrome. It is a reliable source of isoflavones in a convenient beverage format.

I believe that dietary supplements are an ideal form by which individuals can predictably enjoy the health benefits of the health-giving components of soy, particularly isoflavones. However, some individuals continue to insist that the only legitimate way to increase the intake of soy fractions is by increasing soy foods in the diet. The more vociferous critics of supplements have openly criticized their development. But, as I am sure you realize, it is not necessarily practical for busy adults in the West to be meticulous enough about their diets to ensure consistent intake of soy foods, let alone be expected to count isoflavone milligrams. While health-conscious Westerners are adding soy foods to their menus, they are not likely to completely change their food tastes and diets.

The debate about dietary supplements of all types will continue to rage, but this is where I stand on the issue. Soy isoflavones, consumed in supplement form, are among the most significant new "nutriceuticals" available to modern consumers. They have wide-ranging health benefits and are safe at recommended doses. Soy isoflavones are nature's answer to health in the mature female, and increasing evidence indicates that they may have a role in helping to relieve symptoms of PMS.

THE VERSATILE ISOFLAVONES

Soy isoflavones have versatile and potent pharmaceutical effects, and their actions in the body are well-defined. As stated in the previous chapter, isoflavones can exert powerful antioxidant effects and have antiangiogenic activity, which means that they interfere with blood vessel growth, an important cancer-fighting property. Isoflavones are known to inhibit enzymes that promote the growth of several types of cancer. In laboratory experiments, isoflavones have been shown to directly suppress the growth of many types of cancers of human and animal origin. The estrogen-modulating effects of soy isoflavones account for their potential benefit in managing symptoms of menopause, premenstrual syndrome, prostate disease, and estrogen-stimulated cancers. The National Cancer Institute is investing millions of dollars into research studies on soy and cancer, and the Office of Alternative Medicine of the National Institutes of Health is focusing interest in soy and disease prevention and treatment.

I wish to reiterate the hypothesized mode of action of isoflavones as adaptogens in the body. Estrogenic hormones react with nuclear receptors for estrogen in the cells, and their effects on cells and tissues in the body are triggered. Soy isoflavones are capable of binding with these receptors with a different degree of affinity. Picture this as a competition in which the body's estrogenic hormones are competing with isoflavones to attach to the estrogen receptors. When isoflavones attach to the receptors, they can then minimize, or weaken, the effects of the body's estrogen. In other words, in states of estrogen excess, isoflavones exert an antiestrogenic effect by reducing the access of the body's powerful estrogenic hormones to the receptor sites. In contrast, when estrogen is lacking, soy isoflavones are proestrogenic in their action. Thus, isoflavones *modulate* the action of estrogen, and they can be proestrogenic or antiestrogenic, depending on the circumstances of prevailing estrogen dominance. Soy isoflavones have been described as ideal "adaptogens" (compounds that balance functions in the body) by several leading physicians and scientists. In 1997, Dr. Michael B. Schachter, who is one of the nation's leading practitioners of alternative cancer therapy, author of *The Natural Way to a Healthy Prostate*, and President of the Foundation for the Advancement of Innovative Medicine (FAIM) and ACAM, presented several lectures on the adaptogenic activity of soy isoflavones.

Cancer Prevention

Evidence of the protective effects of isoflavones in cancer comes from several sources. Experiments in animals with transplanted tumors, especially tumors dependent on hormonal activity for growth, show that cancer growth is suppressed. There is isolated evidence to the contrary in one recent study in mice with transplanted (foreign) tumors, but it is overwhelmed by many studies that clearly show the anticancer effects of isoflavones.

Some of the strongest and most convincing evidence comes from well-designed population studies that demonstrate the role of soy isoflavones in cancer prevention. Dr. Herman Adlecreutz, physician and professor in the Department of Clinical Chemistry at the University of Helsinki, is a pioneer in this field. He has reviewed many studies and remarked that vegetarians and Asians, who have a low incidence of breast and prostate cancer, are known to excrete high concentrations of phytoestrogens, notably isoflavones. The lower incidence of breast cancer in Singapore and Hong Kong has been directly linked to dietary intake of soy, with isoflavones being the principal agents responsible for the reduced risk. Many other studies of Asian populations also link a lower risk for other types of cancer to their consumption of soy foods.

Reduced risk of prostate cancer among Asian populations has been linked to soy isoflavones in some studies, and other studies imply the same benefit for lung cancer and cancers affecting the gastrointestinal tract. Some scientists are not convinced, however, and continue to argue that population studies are based on observation and do not provide "cast-iron" evidence of a cause-and-effect relationship between soy and cancer prevention. However, this skepticism is rapidly disappearing as evidence accumulates that soy isoflavones have a preventive effect on cancer.

Soy isoflavones exert measurable benefits in cancer prevention, and they have potential for use as therapeutic agents in breast, prostate, and other types of cancer. There is an impressive amount of epidemiological data that supports the potential benefit of soy diet in cancer prevention. These data are supported by an equally impressive series of laboratory experiments that show the anticancer effects of soy-based diets. For example, Dr. Barnes and his colleagues from the University of Alabama showed that modest amounts of soybeans added to the diet of rats caused a 50 percent reduction in breast cancer. The Barnes study, which received considerable media attention, was pivotal in cancer research because it demonstrated unequivocally that soy diets were cancer-protective in animals. The study prompted excitement within the scientific community and precipitated further research in this area.

With some notable exceptions, soy diets have shown cancer-preventive properties in a wide variety of neoplasia (tumor growth) in animals. However, there is always some concern expressed about the portability of animal studies to human circumstances. But, when the epidemiological data are combined with animal data, a convincing body of evidence emerges. There is a good degree of general scientific agreement that soy in various formats is protective against a wide variety of tumors.

There may be complex reasons that occasional studies fail to show the protective benefits of soy. While almost all laboratory animals routinely receive soy-based diets, there are differences in the type of soy food used as well as the processing of the food. For example, soy foods that are processed with solvents tend to lose their valuable isoflavone content. It is probable that the isoflavones, particularly genistein, are the most important anti-cancer agents readily found in certain protein isolates of soy.

An intriguing issue that has received relatively little attention is the fact that soy-based diets are generally used in cancer experiments (using laboratory animals) where anticancer drugs are tested. If most laboratory animals receive soy-based diets, the effects of the diets on the outcome of experiments need to be assessed. However, in many reports of anticancer effects of a variety of drugs or treatments (*i.e.*, cytotoxic drugs, radiotherapy, laser therapy, and so forth), the diet of the animals used in the experiment is not adequately described. Clearly, this is an unrecognized dilemma for cancer researchers. This also means that hundreds of thousands of animal or human experiments exist without such an important consideration as the effect of soy-based diets on disease prevention. Mark and Virginia Messina have noted that no epidemiological studies or animal studies have associated soy diets with enhanced cancer risk. This is highly relevant given the knowledge that many cytotoxic or chemotherapeutic agents that are used in cancer therapy can cause cancer in patients.

It is necessary to reassess results of animal experiments that examined the cancer-preventive role of soy-based diets. Many of these experiments attempt to assess the ability of soy diets to protect an animal against the development of a cancer that is induced by a known, potent carcinogen or carcinogenic process. This type of experimental cancer protection is impressive, but the ability of an agent to protect against spontaneous cancer growth in animals is even more convincing evidence of potential efficacy. In several animal studies, soy-based diets have been shown to be protective against the development of spontaneously occurring breast cancer. Soy-based diets also have been shown to protect against spontaneously occurring liver cancer in mice.

Dava Kava, Ph.D., is an expert on the anticancer effects of soy isoflavones. He points out that genistein in increasing concentrations results in estrogenic effects by creating estrogen-related end products in cells. These "end products" increase at concentrations of genistein similar to those measurable in the blood serum and saliva of people who eat significant amounts of soy foods.

Dr. Kava has looked at cell proliferation in breast tissue. If one places genistein on breast tissue that is estrogen-responsive, then there is an increase in levels of estrogen-related end products. In normal mammary epithelial cells genistein has little effect in small doses, but at higher concentrations of genistein there is a remarkable decrease of cell proliferation due to the cells undergoing a process called apoptosis (a kind of cell arrest and death). In some estrogen receptor positive cells at lower doses, there may be stimulation of growth that is replaced by major inhibition of growth at high concentrations of genistein. In high doses, cell apoptosis and very high levels of inhibition of cell growth occurs with genistein.

The reason proposed is that genistein is acting as an antiestrogen. This is a mechanism of action of isoflavones, proposed by Dr. Mark Messina, which requires reappraisal. Dr. Messina has proposed that genistein acts like the antiestrogen agent Tamoxifen, a drug that is widely used in the treatment of breast cancer. Dr. Kava has presented evidence that genistein is acting as an estrogen agonist (able to combine with a receptor on a cell), not like Tamoxifen. In contrast to estradiol, genistein acts as an estrogen but it decreases cell proliferation, indicating a mechanism of an anticancer effect of genistein that is perhaps unrelated to its actions as an estrogen. These differences of opinion highlight the incomplete nature of the understanding of the biological effects of isoflavones.

The phenolic group of genistein permits it to act as an estrogen, but the double bond of the molecule (hydroxy group 5 hydroxy-keto constituents) on the A and C ring of genistein permits it to act as an antiproliferative agent (meaning that it stops cell division and inhibits cancer growth). The effects of soy isoflavones as anticancer agents seems to be related to non-estrogen-receptor mediated activity. Soy isoflavones interfere with molecules that promote cancer growth, inhibiting the effects of enzymes (protein tyrosine kinase inhibition) and growth factor (epidermal growth factor). They also act as an inhibitor of the growth-regulating enzymes (*e.g.*, DNA topoisamerase), which are responsible for apoptosis. These effects occur at one micromolar to ten micromolar concentrations of genistein. These are concentrations that are achievable with high soy intake or dietary supplementation of soy isoflavones. This complicated dialog merely implies that isoflavones interfere with chemical reactions (enzymes) that promote cancer occurrence and growth.

It appears that genistein is a very good inhibitor of angiogenesis (the growth of new blood vessels). If a cancer cannot develop a blood supply, it will not grow. Genistein interferes with the process of a cancer requiring a blood supply and this antiangiogenic effect is a potent anticancer property of genistein.

Genistein is a good inhibitor of aromatase enzymes and 17 beta hydroxy steroid hydrogenase, which are enzymes that promote the production of estrogens from precursors in the body. It is well-recognized that Asian women living on soy-based diets often have about half the circulating concentrations of estradiol and estrone than Western women not on soy diets.

In summary, genistein and perhaps daidzein may act as pure estrogen agonists, and their anticancer effects (antiproliferative effects) are due to their actions other than their estrogenic effects. Soy isoflavones may just be cancer fighters in disguise. They dress as "women" (estrogen) to get through all the "doors," where they then exert their anticancer effects. Thus they go to an estrogen-receptor positive cell, but act by a host of mechanisms other than an estrogenic effect. Consumption of soy foods or dietary supplements results in soy isoflavones in concentrations that exert important anticancer effects.

SOY AND HEALTHY BONES

Osteoporosis is a common disease among the elderly in Western industrialized countries. Unfortunately, to date there is no safe and effective treatment for this disease once it is well established. The most common type of osteoporosis is associated with bone loss in post-menopausal women. The estrogenic properties of soy isoflavones and some other plant products, such as lignins, have been investigated for their potential to treat and prevent osteoporosis. Based on evidence to date, using isoflavones for this purpose is more than promising.

Several double-blind placebo-controlled clinical trials have shown that semisynthetic isoflavones, notably ipriflavone, are capable of increasing bone density in post-menopausal women. Ipriflavone is approved for use in the treatment of osteoporosis in Europe but not in the United States. When ipriflavone is administered to humans it is converted in part to daidzein, which is a key isoflavone. Here is the irony: Pharmaceutical companies are so intent on protecting their products that they produce ipriflavones to release a soy isoflavone into the body. Does this make sense? Why not give the soy isoflavone daidzein directly?

Important scientific data have emerged from studies conducted by Dr. J. Erdman and his colleagues at the University of Illinois. Their data show unequivocally that the addition of soy protein containing isoflavones can treat osteoporosis by increasing bone density in women with post-menopausal bone loss. This is important because current drugs used to treat osteoporosis—notably, bisphosphonates—have negative side effects. Given the toxicity of bisphosphonates, it is surprising that the medical community is "sleeping" on Dr. Erdman's observations.

ISOFLAVONES AND CARDIOVASCULAR HEALTH

Considerable evidence exists that soy isoflavones can contribute to lowering blood cholesterol levels and inhibit the development of hardening of the arteries (atherosclerosis). The soy isoflavone, genistein, has been shown to directly inhibit several metabolic events that are involved in the cause of atherosclerosis. As for the ability of soy foods to lower cholesterol, over forty studies performed over a period of fifty years form a body of convincing evidence that soy protein containing isoflavones lowers blood

cholesterol very efficiently. James Anderson, M.D., and his colleagues published their work on the cholesterol-lowering effects
of soy in the prominent *New England Journal of Medicine* in
1995, yet the medical profession has been slow to incorporate
these findings into their medical practices. However, conventional practitioners have demonstrated an increasing willingness to
prescribe synthetic lipid-lowering drugs that are fraught with side
effects. The sales of drugs to lower cholesterol are booming while
we forget nutritional interventions for this disorder.

Soy protein, which contains isoflavones, is emerging as a
first-line option for managing high blood cholesterol. I believe it
provides an ideal, safe alternative to the synthetic drugs designed
to lower fats in the blood. In my opinion, synthetic, cholesterol-
lowering drugs are overprescribed, and adverse side effects are
experienced by many individuals taking them. Fortunately, some
physicians are responding to the long-known fact that, along with
lifestyle adjustments, soy protein with isoflavones lowers cholesterol. Genista is a product formulated for this specific purpose.

ANTIOXIDANTS AND ISOFLAVONES

The issue of oxidation and antioxidants currently receives regular
attention in the medical literature and the popular press. The
concern about oxidation can be confusing for consumers because,
inevitably, the term "free radical" enters the picture. Oxidation
occurs when oxygen, obviously a vital element for life, combines
with another substance. Oxidation is an ongoing process in the
body and results from day to day activities such as digesting food,
exercise, or breathing polluted air. During this process, free radicals—unstable molecules—are produced.

The difference between a stable and an unstable molecule
requires an explanation. In a stable molecule electrons are paired,
but during normal physiologic processes, one electron can be lost.
A free radical is a molecule that is missing an electron, making it
highly reactive. The molecule's unpaired electron seeks another
electron, taking it from another cell. This creates another free

radical, and the process starts again. Eventually, the continuous creation of free radicals damages genetic material or membranes in the cells of the body. Free radicals, then, are a by-product of oxidation and are implicated in many of the diseases discussed in this book, including cancer and cardiovascular diseases. Free radicals are also implicated in other conditions associated with aging, such as cataracts and macular degeneration.

When first hearing about free radicals and the damage they can do, many people consider the situation quite bleak; they may feel helpless to do anything about the constant chain of free-radical creation. Since polluted air, tobacco smoke, stress, and even sunlight and exercise—among other things—create free radicals, what is a person to do? Fortunately, nature has created its own natural protection against oxidation and free-radical formation. These protective substances are called antioxidants.

Antioxidant nutrients and compounds protect the body from damage caused by free radicals. Antioxidant substances are abundant in fruit and vegetables, and the isoflavones that are abundant in soybeans are powerful antioxidants. Remember that isoflavones are related to a class of flavonoids, which are potent antioxidants and free-radical scavengers. Soy isoflavones are phenolic compounds, which are cancer-fighting antioxidants. These phytochemicals are called nonnutrient antioxidants. Nutrient antioxidants include vitamins such as C, E, the minerals selenium, copper, manganese, zinc, and other plant compounds, such as those found in green tea.

Until recently, the conventional medical world doubted the importance of antioxidants, but now that their role in preventing many diseases is better understood, the value of antioxidant substances is unquestioned. Looked at as a group, antioxidants comprise a powerful defense system against the potential damage of oxidation and free radical formation.

Each antioxidant has its own action in the body, but the easiest way to view them is as synergistic agents because they work together to protect each other from destruction or damage as a result of oxidation. For example, vitamin C works synergistically with vitamin E, in that vitamin C helps vitamin E regenerate after it has reacted with a free radical. Vitamin E appears to work synergistically with selenium and, in animal studies, supplementing the diet with one of these nutrients relieves the symptoms caused by a deficiency of the other. Soy isoflavones work in a similar manner.

Because antioxidants work together, many health-conscious individuals are attempting to increase foods containing antioxidants and are also taking antioxidants in the form of nutritional supplements. Like other antioxidants, soy isoflavones can be consumed in soy foods or in nutritional supplements.

Epidemiological studies have shown a clear relationship between the consumption of a diet rich in fruits and vegetables and reduced cancer rates. There are also population studies that link soy-based diets with reduced rates of breast, prostate, and colon cancers as well as lower incidence of cardiovascular disease, diabetes, osteoporosis, and so forth. It is clear that soy isoflavones have an important role in protecting the body from the damaging effects of free radicals.

TABLE 2

The basic pathway of antoxidation involves a free radical chain reaction (Bateman et al, 1953). RH $>$ R + H is production of free radical, R is the alkyl radical and RO is the peroxyradical. The peroxyradical can take part in all typical radical-mediated pathways shown as ROO + RH $>$ R + ROOH.

Initiation	RH $>$ R + H
Propagation	R + O $>$ ROO
	ROO + RH $>$ R + ROOH
Termination	R + R
	R + ROO *nonradical products*
	ROO + ROO

NEW ESTROGENS: SERM—
A NEW, BUT NOT SO NEW,
ESTROGEN FORMULATION

In January 1998, the widely read magazine *Your Health* published an article entitled, "New Estrogen: What Every Woman Should Know." Writer Ruth Jacobowitz discussed a new class of drugs that are selective estrogen receptor modulators—or SERMs. This class of drugs mimic estrogen and are being presented to the U.S. Food and Drug Administration (FDA) as an alternative to estrogen replacement therapy (ERT). The approved drug is called raloxifene, produced by Eli Lilly and Company. Given the profit potential of estrogen products, it is not surprising that such a drug has been developed. Ironically, raloxifene is remarkably similar to the action of soy isoflavones, which come with the "small" advantage of thousands of years of safe and effective use.

Raloxifene has commendable properties. It prevents bone loss from the hip and spine and increases bone density. Does it do this as effectively as soy isoflavones? The increase in bone density of 2 to 3 percent with raloxifene may be less than that achievable with soy isoflavones. Raloxifene reduces the so-called "bad" cholesterol (LDL), but so do soy isoflavones. Soy protein with isoflavones increases "good" cholesterol (HDL), but raloxifene does not raise HDL. Raloxifene does not stimulate growth of uterine tissue, and neither do soy isoflavones.

Raloxifene, however, does not help hot flashes, whereas soy isoflavones have been shown, with reasonable consistency, to reduce menopausal symptoms. Perhaps of greater concern is that raloxifene offers no hope to prevent Alzheimer's disease, but estrogen-replacement therapy and perhaps isoflavones do protect against Alzheimer's. (Daidzein, which potentially interacts with estrogen receptors in the brain, may offer such protection.)

These SERMs do not seem to offer anything better than soy isoflavones. But, they are synthetic and can be protected by patents and proprietary interests. Given the choice of a synthetic formulation and natural soy isoflavones, I know which I would choose. When push comes to shove in deciding between estrogenic supplements, SERMs, and soy isoflavones, the natural soy isoflavone supplements appear to win hands down.

THE FAR REACHING HEALTH BENEFITS OF SOY

Since my book *Soya for Health* was published, a great deal of additional information has appeared that supports my assertions that soy foods and soy fractions offer vast health benefits are still largely untapped. Only two or three years ago, many of my colleagues in clinical medicine were skeptical about the wide-ranging potential of soy to improve health and prevent and treat disease. However, I am pleased that many skeptics are changing their minds as evidence keeps pouring in. Soy isoflavones star as among the most interesting, health-giving compounds in the mighty soybean. As you read this book, you will see that isoflavones are only one component of a virtual treasure chest of medicinal and nutrient compounds contained in soybeans.

SOY IS AT THE HEART OF CARDIOVASCULAR WELLNESS

Cardiovascular disease represents a group of conditions that profoundly affects the quality of life of millions of people in the West, particularly the elderly. Soy products have the ability to make a significant contribution in preventing these degenerative conditions that are not only potentially lethal, but rob individuals of their vitality. In some cases, heart disease can be reversed, and soy has a role to play in restoring cardiovascular health. In the next chapter, you will learn how soy foods can help you maintain a healthy heart.

CHAPTER 4

Soy and Your Heart

One of the most important medical developments of our time has been the discovery of a link between high cholesterol levels in the blood and cardiovascular disease. A related discovery, that there is a relationship between high cholesterol levels and a diet high in saturated fat, set the stage for food and diet to become all-important in the campaign to prevent heart disease.

At one time, most of what was known about the heart was discovered by examining the organ during autopsies. When autopsied, heart attack victims, and individuals who died from other causes, were found to have blockages in their arteries. One of the first clues that cholesterol was linked with heart disease came from the discovery that these blockages, referred to as "plaque," contained, among other substances, cholesterol. It was discovered that plaque builds up on the walls of the arteries like mineral deposits in water lines. Evidence indicating that plaque formation was the result of a long, gradual process mounted when autopsies performed on young soldiers in the Korean and Vietnam conflicts revealed that most of these young, presumably healthy men, had at least mild early-stage cholesterol plaque formation. Other research has concluded that even preadolescent children who eat unhealthy diets may have plaque deposits in their coronary arteries. These cholesterol plaques are the forerunners of hardening of the arteries, and they are sometimes called "fatty streaks" in the lining of arterial blood vessels.

At one time, cardiovascular disease was believed to be a genetic issue because Caucasians living in industrialized countries seemed to be afflicted more than any other population group, although other racial groups that moved from their homes to live in the Western world soon developed heart disease, too. The genetic connection, however, seemed like a simple cause-and-effect relationship, and high death rates from heart disease in northern Europe, Canada, and the U.S. were considered unfortunate, but, in large measure, an inevitable consequence of one's genes.

TABLE 3
CORONARY ARTERY DISEASE RISK FACTORS

Established coronary heart disease (CHD) or angina pectoris

Other artherosclerotic disease
      Carotid artery stenosis
      Cerebral vascular disease
      Peripheral vascular disease
      Other occlusive vascular diseases

Cigarette smoking

Hypertension or taking antihypertensive medications

Diabetes mellitus

Low levels of HDL cholesterol (<35 mg/dl)

Family history of premature (CHD) (first-degree relative before age 65)

Severe obesity

Stress, type A personality

Western diet

LOW-FAT DIETS COME OF AGE

It is important to remember that cholesterol is an essential substance for the body, involved in hormone production and other
functions. It enters the bloodstream after being produced by the
liver, as well as entering the bloodstream through food containing
cholesterol, such as eggs and dairy products. Moreover, blood
lipids (lipoproteins), the particles by which cholesterol and other
fats (triglycerides) are carried through the body, are also important. The risk of cardiovascular disease is, in part, measured by
the proportions of different kinds of lipoprotein in the blood—
hence, the common terms "good" and "bad" cholesterol. High-
density lipoprotein (HDL), or "good cholesterol," appears to
protect against heart disease, while low-density lipoprotein
(LDL), or "bad cholesterol," increases the risk of cardiovascular
disease.

THE ESSENTIAL FATTY ACIDS

Any discussion of the so-called good and bad fats in the diet—and
their relationship to a healthy heart and heart disease—must
explore the omega factors, or the essential fatty acids. There are
two important categories of essential fatty acids, the omega-6
series and the omega-3 series. Omega-6 series fatty acids are pervasive in the diet and are found in vegetable foods, whereas
omega-3 fatty acids are primarily found in fish and marine mammals. They are also found in soybeans, which contain significant
fractions of precursors of omega-3 fatty acids.

WHAT DO FATTY ACIDS DO?

One of the most important functions of omega-3 and omega-6
essential fatty acids is to be precursors for hormonal compounds,
especially prostaglandins. Prostaglandins play a major role in
maintaining body structure, function, and homeostasis.

Prostaglandins are needed for and are involved in such critical functions as:

- maintaining normal immune system function;
- hormone production;
- regulating blood pressure;
- regulating responses to pain, inflammation, infection, and cancer;
- controlling the composition and secretions of glands;
- regulating smooth muscle and neural function;
- effecting cell membrane structure and mitosis (a type of cell division);
- regulation of cell oxygenation and nutrient intake; and,
- providing energy substrates for key organs.

As you can see, prostaglandins are essential to health, and necessary fatty acids are essential for the production of prostaglandins. Therefore, announcing that a low-fat diet is beneficial fails to address the critical issue of which types of fat we need and which types we should avoid. Not all dietary fats are bad for health.

Omega-3 Fatty Acids from Plants

The omega-3 family of fatty acids includes alpha-linolenic acid (LNA), eicosopentanoic acid (EPA), and docosahexanoic acid (DHA). Both EPA and DHA can be manufactured by the human body from the essential omega-3 fatty acid LNA (alpha-linolenic acid). This is a slow process, but an important one because LNA is found in several plant foods, including soybeans. EPA and DHA are superunsaturated fatty acids and exert properties that enable them to prevent the buildup of saturated fatty acid deposits in the arteries. Thus, a plant-based diet, such as one that emphasizes soy foods, can be shown by one mechanism to be protective against cardiovascular disease.

However, omega-3 fatty acids found in plants are usually in the form of LNA rather than in the form of EPA and DHA, which is present in fish oil. Several scientists have pointed to the limitations of using omega-3 fatty acids from plant sources because it is believed that there may be many people who are unable to convert LNA into the active constituents EPA and DHA. Proponents of the use of essential fatty acids from plants suggest that this is not a common problem and, if such a problem existed, the body's production of EPA and DHA could be increased simply by increasing the amount of LNA in the diet. The production of EPA and DHA, of course, also promotes the synthesis of "good types" of prostaglandins in the body. Supplemening EPA and DHA exerts powerful health benefits for commoncardiovascular and inflammatory disease.

The fat content of raw soybeans is, on average, about 18 percent. Of that total, about 50 percent of the fat in soy oil is linoleic acid, an omega-6 fatty acid. As much as 8 percent of the fat in soybeans is linolenic acid, an omega-3 fatty acid; about 15 percent is saturated. Therefore, in addition to their other health-promoting benefits, soybean oil represents a source of omega-3 and omega-6 fatty acids. However, this is only true if the soybean oil is in an unrefined state. The heavily processed soybean oil used in the production of commercially packaged food has been turned from a "good" fat into a "bad" fat by being at least partially hydrogenated.

THE PROBLEMS INVOLVED IN DIETARY FAT SOURCES

Methods of processing soybean oil that maintain low temperatures and avoid exposure to light and oxygen generally result in the retention of the essential fatty acid content of the oil, which constitutes its main health-giving fractions. All desirable oils tend to be unrefined and, therefore, free of trans-fatty acids and free radicals. Trans-fatty acids (in contrast to cis-fatty acids) are believed to play a significant role in the promotion of heart disease (and they may also contribute to cancer and diabetes). Unfortunately, most oils available on supermarket shelves are refined oils, and they are generally not suitable for nutriceutical purposes (dietary supplements with predictable health benefits).

If you are interested in obtaining fresh, unrefined soybean oil as a good source of LNA, shop in health food stores or pharmacies. Look for oils that are cold-pressed and unrefined. The labeling of oil products is confusing, so ask the store staff for advice if you need it. Some consumers may assume that "health food" stores carry only healthful types of oil, but this is not necessarily the case. The term "organic," for instance, may be an accurate description of how the original beans from which the oil is extracted were grown, but the oil itself may be refined nonetheless.

WHAT ARE THE NUMBERS?

By midlife, most people expect to have their cholesterol levels checked from time to time. The levels of blood cholesterol and other lipids that can be considered healthy for an individual can only be estimated. However, a good guide to the levels of blood lipids considered healthy is shown in Table 4.

TABLE 4
BLOOD CHOLESTEROL LEVELS AND RISK

	Total Cholesterol	*LDL Cholesterol*
Desirable:	Less than 200 mg/dl	Less than 130 mg/dl
Borderline High Risk:	200 - 239 mg/dl	130-159 mg/dl
High Risk:	Greater than 240 mg/dl	Greater than 160 mg/dl

cholesterol levels was proposed by the adult treatment of the National Cholesterol Education Program

This cholesterol "counting" system is not foolproof. Some individuals with high cholesterol may live a long, healthy life, while some individuals with low cholesterol may die prematurely. However, it is known that the overall average range of total blood cholesterol levels of adult Americans and western Europeans is 210–225 mg/dl, and statistical studies demonstrate with clarity that the death rate from coronary artery disease increases if blood cholesterol levels increase. When the blood cholesterol level is 240 mg/dl, the mortality rate from cardiovascular diseases increases four-fold above the average rate; at 260 mg/dl, the risk of death is six-fold or greater.

Total cholesterol is not the only measure of risk. The ratio of HDL to LDL is another reasonable measure of coronary artery disease risk, as is the ratio between HDL and total cholesterol. The desirable ratio of HDL to LDL is one that favors a preponderance of HDL. Ratios can be confusing, however. For example, looking at ratios of total cholesterol to HDL leads to a desirable ratio of less than 4.5. The ratio can be altered by raising LDL or lowering HDL, which tends to push the ratio higher, in contrast to lowering LDL and raising HDL, which tends to push the ratio lower.

It is easy to become obsessed with cholesterol numbers. A healthy adult would ideally have a blood cholesterol range in the 120–180 mg/dl, but under 200 is often regarded as quite acceptable. In any event, there is little point in having a blood cholesterol of 120 mg/dl and continuing to smoke, drink excessively, and lead a sedentary lifestyle.

DIET AND DIETARY CONSTITUENTS LOWER CHOLESTEROL

The lipid, or hypercholesterolemic, theory of coronary heart disease is not characterized by simple cause-and-effect relationships. In my opinion, the reason for this is that the disease involves multiple causes, not because high blood cholesterol is unimportant. Cholesterol, after all, is an essential component of the human body, and it is an important precursor for the manufacture of sex hormones, other steroid hormones, and bile acids in the human body. It is often forgotten that blood cholesterol levels fluctuate, and some studies indicate that blood cholesterol levels tend to be higher during the winter months than during the summer months.

Modern research also indicates that the synthesis of cholesterol by the human body must be recognized as equally, if not more, important than dietary intake of cholesterol in several circumstances. It is known, for instance, that in the absence of dietary cholesterol the synthesis of cholesterol by the body is similar in individuals with either high or low blood cholesterol. Furthermore, variability in certain people's responses to their own synthesis or utilization of cholesterol are affected by dietary intake of cholesterol. Dietary cholesterol has been observed to actually interrupt cholesterol synthesis by the body.

Added to these facts from recent research on cholesterol synthesis, there is now increasing recognition that a diet high in animal protein and saturated fat generally leads to higher blood cholesterol levels and, by inference, more atherosclerosis than a diet of plant protein. The Council for Agricultural Science and Technology (CAST) in the U.S. has acknowledged the potential importance of plant protein in causing lower cholesterol levels. It is important to note at this point that saturated fat in the diet is more atherogenic than unsaturated fat, regardless of the cholesterol content of the diet. Saturated fat often contributes more to raising blood cholesterol than does excessive dietary intake of cholesterol. Thus, consuming soy protein in the diet, with appropriate reductions of saturated fat and cholesterol, represents an ideal pathway to lower cholesterol levels and prevention of heart disease. I believe that this is a first-line option for fighting coronary artery disease, given the overwhelming amount of cumulative evidence that soy protein in daily doses of 25 grams or more lowers cholesterol. In my opinion, the consumption of soy, in many circumstances, obviates the need for prescription drugs to lower blood cholesterol.

DRUGS TO THE RESCUE?

In recent years, drugs to lower cholesterol have been viewed erroneously as a panacea for reducing the risk of high blood cholesterol and plaque buildup in the arteries. It is true that there are powerful drugs that do, indeed, lower cholesterol, at least some of the time. The question remains, however, at what cost—or costs—do these drugs work? First, the side effects experienced by some people are unpleasant at best, and dangerous at worst, with the risks ranging from abdominal pain and nausea to liver damage. Too, the drugs are very expensive—well over a hundred dollars a month! It is no wonder researchers and the general public are looking for a safer solution to the cholesterol problem.

The Short-Sighted Solution

Therapy that is targeted to just lower cholesterol is shortsighted or even foolish medicine. Lowering cholesterol by using a synthetic lipid-lowering drug without including a nutritional program to improve general health is neither safe nor cost-effective. Nutritional programs that reduce cholesterol are generally safer and often cheaper than drug therapy, and they add an advantage seldom brought up in drug therapy—the advantage of promoting overall wellness.

SOY MAY BE THE HEART'S FRIEND

There is overwhelming evidence that soy protein lowers cholesterol levels in the blood. Epidemiological studies—that is, studies across populations—supports this conclusion. The studies indicate that cultures that rely primarily on vegetable protein rather than animal protein have lower incidence of cardiovascular diseases, a lower prevalence of elevated blood pressure (hypertension), and less atherosclerosis (arterial blockages). Asian cultures in particular have a much lower death rate from cardiovascular diseases and, of course, we now know that soy is an important source of protein for diets in many Asian countries.

We do not have to rely just on population studies. Animal studies first showed that soy protein could lower cholesterol in the blood and, because soy is inherently safe (not to mention inexpensive) research protocols involving humans were not slow in coming. The result is that many studies on humans exist. In one, patients with elevated cholesterol showed an average reduction of 21 percent in blood serum levels after only three weeks on a diet in which animal protein was replaced with soy protein. The soy regimen also outpaced a parallel group placed on a standard low-fat diet that included some animal protein. Other studies have shown that if we want to reduce cholesterol levels quickly, using soy protein is a safe, inexpensive, and effective way to proceed.

DR. JAMES ANDERSON'S BREAKTHROUGH WORK

Dr. James Anderson of the University of Kentucky has demonstrated in his 1995 article in the *New England Journal of Medicine* that many studies indicate that soy protein lowers cholesterol. Dr. Anderson analyzed thirty-eight reports of clinical studies, and his review of these studies show substantial reductions of blood cholesterol by soy protein supplementation or switching to soy protein in the diet. It should be noted that the reductions in blood cholesterol and lipids are similar to those achieved with maintenance doses of synthetic pharmaceuticals.

Dr. Anderson's soy study has had a major impact on conventional and alternative medical practices. Anderson and his colleagues have traced work that demonstrates that vegetable protein in the diet, as a replacement for animal protein, appears to be associated with a lower risk of coronary artery disease. The major reason for this finding relates to the ability of vegetable-based diets, particularly soy-based diets, to lower blood cholesterol.

After analyzing the studies, Dr. Anderson and his colleagues have conclusively shown that consumption of soy protein-containing isoflavones in the diet, in contrast to animal protein, significantly decreases blood levels of total cholesterol, LDL cholesterol, and triglycerides. Soy exerts beneficial effects by increasing the "good" HDL cholesterol.

The most important finding of Dr. Anderson's study was that decreases in serum cholesterol were noted in a manner that appeared to be independent of any major changes in body weight. Soy protein isolates have a clear advantage over drug therapy and should be offered, along with a low-cholesterol dietary plan, as the initial treatment for high cholesterol.

HOW DOES SOY LOWER CHOLESTEROL?

The exact mechanism of soy's ability to lower blood cholesterol is not fully known, but that is not unusual in science, as you no doubt know. We can postulate any number of reasons for soy's protective action, among them the fact that its isoflavone content makes it an effective antioxidant, meaning that it can protect the walls of the arteries from damage by free radicals. Isoflavones inhibit the oxidation of LDL, and oxidized LDL is the form of cholesterol that is often found in the plaque that causes atherosclerosis. Other nutrients are also known to have similar effects. Vitamin E, another antioxidant, is also considered effective against plaque buildup. Once scoffed at, vitamin E is now part of the treatment protocol for patients who have had bypass surgery. I would go one further and add soy to the diet of these individuals.

We could also examine the amino acid composition of soy protein. In February of 1998, researchers identified the amino acid homocysteine as associated with an increased risk of cardio-vascular disease. One of the specific agents for making homo-cysteine harmless is the amino acid glycine, which soy protein contains in abundance. In general, increases of arginine and glycine are associated with decreases in serum cholesterol; soy protein is rich in both arginine and glycine. In addition, animal protein is proportionately lower in these amino acids, but is higher in lysine, which raises insulin levels and promotes cholesterol synthesis—or production—in the liver.

Of all the suggested mechanisms for the cholesterol-lowering effect of soy protein, Dr. Kenneth Setchell, a professor at the Children's Hospital Medical Center in Cincinnati, Ohio, believes that it is the isoflavones in soy that contribute most to its lipid-lowering effects. The rationale for implicating soy estrogens as cholesterol-lowering agents comes from experiments in which the administration of oral estrogens, or the synthetic weak estrogen tamoxifen, can be shown to decrease both serum LDL and cholesterol levels. It has been proposed that isoflavones in soy are capable of similar actions to those that occur with oral estrogens and tamoxifen. However, I do not recommend estrogen-replacement therapy or tamoxifen as a way to lower cholesterol.

Very interesting studies in monkeys show that soy isoflavones account for up to three quarters of the measurable effect of lowering blood cholesterol. If soy protein that is lacking in isoflavones is fed to primates, blood cholesterol is not reduced, but when soy protein containing isoflavone is given, blood cholesterol is lowered. Monkeys are the closest animal model to humans and, therefore, the results of these experiments appear to have definite relevance to the observed human effects of a diet supplemented with soy protein containing isoflavones. Several other studies provide corroborating evidence of the ability of soy protein containing isoflavones to lower blood cholesterol. In one study, adding isoflavones to the diet was found to cause blood cholesterol to fall by as much as 35 percent.

It is ironic that only a few years ago, criticism was directed at the medical establishment for its tendency to ignore the risk of heart disease among postmenopausal women. Not only were many drug trials restricted to male research subjects, but women were less likely to be screened for developing cardiovascular conditions. The criticism was well-founded, but the solution to the problem is misguided. Over the last two or three years, women's magazines and other media reports directed to women are dominated with data promoting cholesterol-lowering drugs. Rarely, if ever, is adding soy to the diet mentioned as an option for preventing heart disease or lowering cholesterol levels. This is strange, given the overwhelming evidence that soy is beneficial in the menopausal female.

Estrogen, an important reproductive hormone, is believed to have a protective mechanism for heart disease, which is one of the reasons women are urged to take estrogen during and following menopause. The plant estrogens found in soybeans may offer similar benefits. These are "weak" estrogens, meaning they do not have the potential to stimulate hormonally dependent cancers, but they may be one key to soy's protective effect on the heart.

OTHER BENEFITS OF SOY FOR YOUR HEART

Along with isoflavones, several components of soybeans other than protein may have a cholesterol-lowering effect, including fiber, phytosterols, saponins, and lecithin. Lecithin has been touted repeatedly as a cholesterol-lowering agent, and it has enjoyed considerable use in a relatively purified format for the reduction of blood cholesterol. However, the relatively large amounts of lecithin required to reduce cholesterol, and the real concerns about its efficacy in fighting cholesterol, keep its use limited.

Fiber contained within soybeans can lower blood cholesterol, and it shares this lipid-lowering effect with many different types of dietary fiber. Total dietary intake is important in maintaining good health, and other efficient sources of fiber include bran, oats, and other grains that are not overly refined. Several well-conducted studies in humans indicate that fiber derived from soy will effectively lower blood cholesterol. Soy fiber has been very underestimated as a potential, safe lipid-lowering agent in humans.

Saponins found in soy products may also act to lower blood cholesterol. Saponins bear a chemical similarity to cholesterol and may either block the absorption of cholesterol or enhance its excretion.

WHAT OPTIONS DO YOU HAVE?

Researchers and clinicians such as Dean Ornish, M.D.—director of the Preventive Medicine Research Institute, an official physician to President Clinton, and consultant to the White House chefs since 1993—have demonstrated that a low-fat, vegetarian diet, combined with lifestyle modifications, have positive benefits for both the prevention and treatment of heart disease. Practicing yoga, regular walking, and engaging in meditation, which are components of Dr. Ornish's Program for Reversing Heart Disease, are valuable regardless of one's age or health status. Dr. Ornish's Program is medically and philosophically sound, and produces positive results. The question is, of course, will you—or can you—incorporate all these elements into your life? For many busy Westerners, the answer is no. Among many health-conscious people, a regular exercise program and periodic attempts to reduce stress is about all they can handle.

Being obsessively vigilant about diet is also not easy for most people, but one can start by gradually substituting soy products for animal protein and by reducing overall fat. The amount of soy protein necessary to reduce an already high cholesterol level is relatively modest. Replacing approximately half the animal protein intake in a normal diet with soy protein can significantly reduce LDL cholesterol. Studies have indicated that the addition of 20 to 25 grams of soy protein to the daily diet is effective at reducing cholesterol in most people.

WHAT DO BLOOD PRESSURE READINGS INDICATE?

Blood pressure measurements are expressed in two values: systolic pressure, which is maximum pressure reached as the blood surges into the arteries during physical exertion; and diastolic pressure, which is the lowest point to which the pressure drops. It is the diastolic, or resting blood pressure, that is used to determine whether the condition called chronic hypertension is present. (The term "resting" is not meant to imply that you are asleep or have been sitting quietly for a long period of time. It simply means that you are seated and are not involved in intense physical activity.) A reading of 110 (systolic) over 70 (diastolic) is considered a favorable reading for an adult. The normal range is defined as a systolic reading of 140 or below and a diastolic reading of 85 and below. A reading of 140–150 (systolic) over 85–89 (diastolic) is the high-normal range. Readings of 150 over 90 or higher are indicative of hypertension, with some adjustment made for older adults, for whom 150/90 might be a reading that falls into a normal range.

Because hypertension is silent, in that it produces no outward symptoms, and because its consequences are serious, it is considered a "silent killer"—a primary cause of premature death in the West. Nearly two million people are diagnosed with the condition annually and, in the vast majority of cases, the cause is not linked with other medical conditions. About 25 percent of the adult population of the U.S. is at risk for a disease that has the potential to cause premature death. The key to solving the problem of hypertension is prevention. A healthful lifestyle, including maintaining a normal weight, exercising regularly, and managing stress are probably the best preventive measures you can implement.

SOY HAS A ROLE TO PLAY

The lifestyle risk factors for high blood pressure are similar to those for coronary artery disease. In addition, hypertension is itself a risk factor for developing cardiovascular diseases, so prevention for both conditions tends to include similar recommendations. While a soy-based diet cannot eliminate risk factors such as smoking or a sedentary lifestyle, it can offer beneficial dietary modifications that promote cardiovascular health. To begin with, vegetarians tend to have lower blood pressure than those who use animal protein as the mainstay of their diets.

Japanese researchers have shown that fermented soy foods, such as nato and miso, contain antihypertensive peptides (chains of amino acids occurring in a specific sequence) that appear to interfere with an enzyme (angiotensin-converting enzyme) that promotes a chemical (angiotensin) which, in turn, elevates blood pressure. What is remarkable about this is that many of the medications used in standard medical practice attempt to block the same enzyme.

The amino acid content of soy protein is considered key to another way it appears to control blood pressure. Soy protein's lower content of sulphur-containing amino acids fosters greater excretion of salt and less excretion of calcium through the kidneys. Calcium, a mineral well-known for its value in building and maintaining the health of the bones and teeth, appears also to play a role in regulating blood pressure. Several studies have demonstrated that supplementing the diet with calcium results in small but significant reductions in blood pressure in those with mild to moderate disease. Calcium supplements may also aid in reducing blood cholesterol and triglycerides.

SUMMING UP ON SOY

Many popular magazines, newspapers, and consumer books highlight growing concerns about cardiovascular disease, the number-one killer and cause of premature death in Western nations. Many of these same publications feature reports about the health benefits of soybeans. However, it is apparent that the average person will not be able to consume the amount of health-giving fractions of soybeans that are required to achieve an optimum health benefit. In my opinion, the judicious use of dietary soy supplements is emerging as a first-line option in the treatment and prevention of heart disease.

There is a switch going on in our attitudes toward diet, away from an emphasis on animal protein to an emphasis on vegetable protein. One of the major risk factors for cardiovascular disease is obesity. In the next chapter, I will discuss the ways in which soy can be of benefit in the fight against this major disease of Western societies.

CHAPTER 5

Soy and Weight Control

The phrase, "diets don't work," is popular today at least in part because it expresses sentiments that reflect the experiences of many dieters. Unfortunately the statement is not completely accurate. In fact, while many weight loss diets do not work, one's *diet* is still certainly an important part of the problem of being overweight. It is generally true that if you eat too much you will be fat, and if you do not eat enough you will be thin. Look at it this way: "energy in"—food—has to be balanced by "energy out"—exercise and body metabolism. This is not the whole story, but many a quack or charlatan wants you to ignore this basic law of thermodynamics.

OBESITY VERSUS OVERWEIGHT

Defining obesity precisely is a difficult task. True obesity is a medical condition and is defined as being more than 20 percent above ideal body weight. Using this definition, about 25 percent of the U.S. population is obese. More alarming, however, is that at least one in three individuals has a degree of overweight that puts them at *some* medical risk. As the general public becomes more aware of the risks of obesity, overweight individuals are becoming increasingly worried about their health.

Table 5 lists conditions in which being overweight or obesity is a contributing factor. Some of these diseases are discussed in detail in this book because adding soy to the diet has been shown to be effective as part of a prevention program for them. However, even if this were not true, soy's nutrition profile alone would be enough to put it at the basis of a healthful weight control plan.

THE VERY FAT PERSON

Morbid obesity, usually defined as being 50 to 100 percent above desirable body weight, is the most serious condition related to being overweight. Major obesity affects approximately two million adults between the ages of twenty and seventy-nine. Cardiovascular disease, diabetes mellitus, kidney disorders, arthritis, and other chronic diseases are often present in the obese, especially when obesity has been present for many years.

TABLE 5
RISKS AND COMPLICATIONS OF OBESITY

Glucose intolerance°
Diabetes mellitus°
Hypertension°
Hypercholesterolemia°
Cardiac disease: atherosclerotic disease, congestive heart failure
Pulmonary disease: sleep apnea, chronic lung disease
Cerebrovascular disease, stroke°
Cancer: breast, uterus, colon, prostate°
Gallbladder: stones°
Pregnancy risks
Surgery risks
Renal failure
Gout
Infertility
Degenerative arthritis°
Early death
Psychological problems: poor self image
Social problems: discrimination in jobs, education, and marriage

°Complications of obesity that are amenable to corrections by soy-based diets.

Morbid obesity aside, most adults—and a growing number of children and adolescents—are concerned about becoming overweight and having to face the increased risk of developing the degenerative diseases listed in Table 5. Health conscious individuals wisely view the maintenance of an ideal weight as a kind of insurance policy against future illness. However, the question: "What is an ideal weight?" should be changed to the question: "What is the ideal weight range?" with several numbers falling in that ideal range.

While people have the right to object to an assessment of their health based on numbers on a scale, the Metropolitan Height and Weight Tables, updated in 1983, do provide useful guidelines (See Table 6).

Having a notion that there is one ideal weight, or body type, can help motivate a person to work toward a goal, but it can also contribute to a self-defeating state that results in failure to lose weight. Therefore, I think it is important for people to be comfortable with gradual-loss regimens and even modest shedding of pounds, especially if they can sustain their weight loss. The overweight person who imagines the body image of models such as Kate Moss is often disappointed.

How Many Pounds, and Where Are They Located?

Recently, considerable attention has been given to the phenomenon of distribution of body fat. Measuring the minimal circumference of the waist and the maximum circumference of the hips (waist-to-hip ratio, or WHR) helps define obesity in terms of the distribution of upper or lower body fat. In general, individuals whose excess body fat is carried in the upper body—the back of the neck, shoulder areas, and inner abdomen—appear to be at higher risk for cardiovascular disease, hypertension, diabetes, and some forms of cancer in comparison with individuals whose excess pounds are carried in the hips and buttocks. A few years ago, the risk of heart disease in women was described as greater for the "apple-shaped" woman than for the "pear-shaped" woman.

TABLE 6
METROPOLITAN LIFE INSURANCE COMPANY'S
MEN'S HEIGHT AND WEIGHT TABLES (1996)

Height (ft/in)*	Weight (lbs)*		
	Small Frame	Medium Frame	Large Frame
5'2"	128-134	131-141	138-150
5'3"	130-136	133-143	140-153
5'4"	132-138	135-145	142-156
5'5"	134-140	137-148	144-160
5'6"	136-142	139-151	146-164
5'7"	138-145	142-154	149-168
5'8"	140-148	145-157	152-172
5'9"	142-151	148-160	155-176
5'10"	144-154	151-163	158-180
5'11"	146-157	154-166	161-184
6'0"	149-160	157-170	164-188
6'1"	152-164	160-174	168-192
6'2"	155-168	164-178	172-197
6'3"	158-172	167-182	176-202
6'4"	162-176	171-187	181-207

METROPOLITAN LIFE INSURANCE COMPANY'S
WOMEN'S HEIGHT AND WEIGHT TABLES (1996)

4'10"	102-111	109-121	118-131
4'11"	103-113	111-123	120-134
5'0"	104-115	113-126	122-137
5'1"	106-118	115-129	125-140
5'2"	108-121	118-132	128-143
5'3"	111-124	121-135	131-147
5'4"	114-127	124-138	134-151
5'5"	117-130	127-141	137-155
5'6"	120-133	130-144	140-159
5'7"	123-136	133-147	143-163
5'8"	126-139	136-150	146-167
5'9"	129-142	139-153	149-170
5'10"	132-145	142-156	152-173
5'11"	135-148	145-159	155-176
6'0"	138-151	148-162	158-179

*Weights for adults age 25-59 years based on lowest mortality. Weight in pounds according to frame size wearing indoor clothing (5 pounds for men and 3 pounds for women) and shoes with one-inch heels.

Through simple observation, most people can determine which "form of fruit" their body most resembles. However, if you want to be certain, simply measure your waist at its smallest point and measure your hips at their widest point. Then divide your waist measurement by your hip measurement. A result that is less than 0.75 means that you are "pear-shaped"; a ratio greater than 0.80 puts you in the very "apple-shaped" range.

Awareness of this connection between fat distribution and your health could be used to your advantage in the design of your exercise program. For example, in recent years greater numbers of women have engaged in weight training designed to build muscle tissue in the upper body. This activity not only increases strength, but it can also assist in reducing fat tissue in the upper area of the body.

Calculating percentages of body fat and distribution must always take into account the physiological differences between males and females. By nature's design, a healthy woman will have a larger percentage of body fat than a healthy man. In fact, when a woman does not have adequate body fat, she may stop menstruating and her body may not be able to support a pregnancy.

How Did Obesity Become So Prevalent?

There are many reasons for the widespread problem of being overweight. Certainly a genetic component has to be included among the causes. About 25 percent of all children are overweight, and they generally come from families in which the adults are overweight. In fact, about 25 percent of all adults are overweight, too. However, being predisposed to a condition does *not* mean that one is doomed to develop it or cannot take measures to control it.

Without doubt, faulty eating patterns and habits contribute to weight gain. Fat- and sugar-laden foods are staple items in the pantries of many families, and few of us are immune to television commercials or other media advertising that encourage us to reward ourselves with rich desserts and unending indulgence in snack food. Convenience foods in supermarkets have changed the way people select the food they eat, and working parents find they have to substitute fast-food restaurants for the task of preparing meals at home every day. Fatty foods taste good, and they are satisfying. Unfortunately, the tastes acquired in childhood are difficult to overcome as adults.

Dangers of High-Fat Diet in Childhood

In his book, *Dr. Attwood's Low-fat Prescription For Kids*, pediatrician Charles R. Attwood has raised a warning flag for parents about the relationship between diet in childhood and the chances of developing heart disease in later life. According to Dr. Attwood, the fat habit, while not easy to alter, can be phased out. In his book, he offers a four-stage plan to reduce fat in the daily diet so that children—and the adults following the plan with them—will lose their preference for it. Eating high-fat foods creates a craving for more of these foods. Therefore, avoiding them eliminates the craving. In other words, if children and adults develop a taste for low-fat food, that becomes the new habit. Eventually, fatty meats and whole milk, for example, have no appeal.

Gaining and Losing and Gaining Again

The phenomenon of "yo-yo" dieting—cycles of rapid weight loss and gain—are believed to be associated with very significant health risks. Men and women who have experienced the weight gain that often follows a diet in which daily calorie intake is below 1,200 calories can vouch for the fact that a rebound weight gain is sure to follow when "normal" eating is resumed. The rebound weight gain that follows calorie restriction is explained by a correction the body's metabolism makes to accommodate the original low-calorie intake. This accommodation does not rapidly reverse.

Therefore, when the desired weight is reached (or at whatever point the person stops the diet), the metabolic rate in effect remains the same as it was when the body was heavier. Quite logically, weight gain results, often bringing a sense of hopelessness to the person trying to diet.

Individuals can only overcome the yo-yo effect if they engage in behavior modification while they diet and understand that maintaining weight loss must be viewed as a long-term commitment. The lesson is, if you want to lose weight permanently, lose it slowly.

As a general principle, I also reject the notion of ideal weight. A person with a history of obesity will rarely achieve a so-called ideal weight. The acceptable and sound compromise is to attempt to return to a healthful weight range. This is important, because overweight individuals will often fail to achieve optimal weight reduction if they set unreasonable goals for themselves. If someone has been more than 20 percent above an ideal weight for a significant period of time, then dieting with a goal to look like a fashion model is self-defeating.

SOY AND WEIGHT LOSS

It is important to remember that obesity is not a universal problem, equally affecting all societies. In a study of dietary habits and obesity among men from seven countries, Japanese men had, by far, the lowest rate of obesity (Table 7). It is no coincidence that the diets of the Japanese are, in general, "plant-based" and low in fat. More specifically, they include generous amounts of soy foods and fiber.

With or without exercise, or even prescription medications, permanent changes in diet will always be the cornerstone of any weight-loss program whose effects have at least a chance of being lasting. Soy is a perfect nutrient for this type of permanent weight-loss diet. It is low in calories, low in fat, and very nutritious.

I recommend the following elements of a holistic approach to losing weight, or maintaining an ideal weight. This program

TABLE 7
PREVALENCE OF OVERWEIGHT AND OBESITY
IN MEN FROM SEVEN COUNTRIES*

| Country | Percent of sample | |
	Overweight	Obese
Italy	33	28
United States	32	63
Yugoslavia	19	29
Finland	15	14
Netherlands	13	32
Greece	11	11
Japan	2	2

*From Keys (1970)

should be carried out under the supervision of a health care provider.

- **A primarily plant-based diet**, of which soy is a basic component. The protein content of soy makes it a good substitute across the board for most animal protein, including dairy products. Many soy products are also relatively low in fat to begin with, and they often have their fat content further reduced in the production process. For example, reduced-fat soy milk and tofu are readily available in health food stores and some mainstream supermarkets.

  In addition, soy foods contain beneficial types of fats, such as omega-3 and omega 6-fatty acids. Soy in the form of texturized vegetable protein is available as a substitute for meat or poultry. Because it is filling and satisfying, rich in the basic nutrients—protein, carbohydrate, and fat—and comes in a great variety of forms, soy truly is the perfect dieter's food.

- **An exercise program** that is manageable and not beyond your physical limits. Just about everyone can undertake a walking program. Many books and videotapes are available to help you begin a sensible walking program that gradually increases both the pace and the distance covered. If you need to lose a moderate amount of weight, it is likely that no special instruction is needed. However, obese individuals should seek help from a physician in collaboration with a qualified exercise instructor. Many overweight individuals simply will not exercise in a health club or in any public place. Fortunately, exercise can be performed in the privacy of your home.

- **Psychological support** is essential for many overweight individuals, especially for those who have long believed that they are weak-willed and flawed. While I realize that many overweight men and women lead full and productive lives, most will admit that their weight difficulties take a toll.

    Support can be found in the form of groups or through individual counseling, and this is a component of treatment that should not be overlooked. It is also absolutely necessary to modify eating behaviors and attitudes toward food in order to avoid regaining weight after the desired weight is reached. Learning the principles of behavior modification is necessary for a nutrition and lifestyle program that works.

- **Nutritional education** is also critical, particularly when making permanent dietary changes. While it may not be necessary to become a strict vegetarian, a diet rich in soy and other plant foods usually requires adjusting to a new way of eating and cooking. The fact is, a low-fat diet is optimal for the whole family, but if this is not possible, it may be necessary for the dieter in the family to eat differently from the rest of the family. While I know this is a difficult undertaking for many people, in the long-run it will be worth it.

    Equally important to remember is that few people should consume less than 1200 calories a day on a self-imposed diet to lose weight. This is a well-accepted minimum.

Currently, calorie counting is not as popular as weighing and measuring food in order to gain control over the size of the portions. Eliminating excess fat in the diet is a first step to lowering the number of total calories consumed.

Soy Promotes Overall Health with Weight Loss

Readily available, low in fat, high in nutrients and fiber, soy foods are an all-but-perfect food for achieving weight loss. The many other health benefits they confer make them indispensible. For example, it has been well-established that the addition of soy protein containing isoflavones to the diet lowers blood cholesterol. Add to that the fact that the fatty acids in soy are beneficial to the cardiovascular system in comparison to other types of fat, and you have what is popularly known today as a "heart-smart" food. Soy foods also help prevent some serious diseases such as osteoporosis and cancer. In short, making soy foods a significant element in your diet promotes health in a major way. During the process of weight loss, unhealthy things may happen. Calcium can be lost from bones, lean muscle mass can be reduced, and gallstones may form. Soy can reverse these untoward effects of weight loss by conserving body calcium, promoting muscle health, and interfering with gallstone formation.

Because the consequences of overweight are serious, I believe that we should view this as a serious public health concern. We are fooling ourselves if we believe we can solve the problem without a fundamental change in dietary habits. As an individual, your immediate goal may be to lose weight, but your long-term goal must be to maintain a weight that is right for you and to build your health. Soy foods can help you reach both goals.

CHAPTER 6

Soy and Diabetes Mellitus

Diabetes mellitus is a degenerative disease of unknown cause that is common in Western society. The symptoms of the disease result from a deficiency in the amount of insulin produced by the pancreas. Insulin is mandatory for moving glucose (sugar), the body's principal energy source, into the cells, or into the liver and fat cells where it is stored. Glucose is the source of energy for every living cell in the body, so an interruption in this system has critical consequences. If the pancreas is unable to produce sufficient insulin—or any insulin—then glucose levels rise. A lack of insulin means that the body is unable to use, or store, this glucose, which means that the body's cells are deprived of their energy source. Fatigue, excessive thirst, and frequent urination are common symptoms of diabetes mellitus. Blurred vision, frequent urinary tract infections, and, in women, recurring vaginal yeast infections, are also signs that diabetes may have developed.

There are at least two types of diabetes mellitus. In type I, or juvenile-onset diabetes, the insulin-secreting cells in the pancreas have been destroyed, making the body unable to produce insulin. Once this happens, the need for insulin injections is generally absolute. It is proposed that many cases of type I diabetes develop as a result of a viral infection that causes an immune response, which destroys the cells in the pancreas (islets of Langerhans, or pancreatic cell clusters) that secrete insulin. In any case, the onset of type I diabetes is often rapid and the condition is permanent. Individuals with type I diabetes are usually followed closely by a primary care physician, but proper diet is also critical for their overall health and well-being.

Type II diabetes is more prevalent than type I. Often called maturity-onset diabetes, it strikes adults—especially older adults—and, unlike type I diabetes, it generally progresses slowly. Type II diabetes is a degenerative disease, meaning that the body gradually produces less insulin, or the insulin being produced cannot be used because the cell receptors for insulin gradually cease to respond to the hormone.

Obesity is a primary risk factor for type II diabetes mellitus because excess weight—specifically, excess fat—greatly increases the body's demands for insulin. In overweight individuals, the cells are also less sensitive to insulin, which means sufficient insulin may be produced but it cannot be efficiently used. Approximately 75 percent of Type II diabetics are overweight. There is an inherited tendency to both obesity and to diabetes, but a predisposition to a disease does not mean that an individual will develop it. Preventive measures can still make a difference. Type II diabetes in an overweight person can sometimes be reversed when the patient achieves a normal weight. Dietary modification and lifestyle improvement also can reverse type II diabetes in people with normal weight.

SPOTTING DIABETES

Type II diabetes is frequently silent in its early stages and is often discovered during a routine medical exam. Most frequently, the disease does not produce severe symptoms. However, even if no symptoms appear, diabetes is still capable of inflicting long-term damage to many organs in the body, particularly the eyes, kidneys, heart, and cardiovascular system. Diabetes also threatens eyesight by causing proliferation of the blood vessels surrounding the retina (the light-sensitive area in the back of the eye). Atherosclerosis, a common complication of diabetes, may cause decreased circulation to the extremities. Poor circulation, in turn, is associated with peripheral nerve damage (neuropathy) and with serious conditions of the feet, including ulcers and the loss of toes.

INADEQUATE DIETS ENTER THE PICTURE

Diabetes is regarded by some as the oldest nutritional deficiency disease. For a hundred years, physicians have suspected that it is induced by refined diets, which are by definition low in fiber. It is probably no exaggeration to claim that the current prevalence of diabetes is one of the results of Western affluence. Over time, whole grains, beans, and legumes came to be regarded as the diet of the poor, while being rich meant you could afford highly refined and processed grains, sugar-rich and fat-laden prepared foods, and meals centered around meat and poultry. As affluence has spread, this refined diet has become the norm, now making nearly everyone at risk for diabetes. Recent statistics from the American Diabetes Association show a galloping increase in new cases of diabetes.

Diabetes ranks as the seventh leading cause of death in the United States. Even that ranking is deceptive because diabetes mellitus contributes to kidney failure and cardiovascular disease, and its presence increases the risk of stroke. In addition, the majority of cases of new blindness in Western societies are attributable to diabetes. In other words, the disease can lead to serious and life-threatening damage to vital organs and systems in the body. Even with increased knowledge about the treatment of diabetes mellitus, life expectancy is considerably lower among diabetics than among nondiabetics.

This situation is improving, however, and in my opinion, can further improve with the use of soy. Diabetes mellitus is a classic example of a disease where diligent self-care promotes well-being. In many ways, diabetics are the most health-conscious among us because the consequences of mismanaging their disease may be potentially life-threatening and, at the very least, seriously degrade their quality of life. Because diet is the most critical area for self-care of the disease, it makes good sense to plan the best diet possible, and the best diet includes soy foods. It is my opinion that soy foods offer significant benefits in both the prevention and treatment of diabetes. The use of soy-based diets is one of the most overlooked, simple measures that could make a major contribution to the health and well-being of people with diabetes mellitus!

Carbohydrates and Diabetes

A diabetic's focus on the effects of carbohydrate intake must include the important fact that all carbohydrates are not of equal value. Simple carbohydrates are contained mainly in foods that are highly refined and generally stripped of their naturally occurring fiber. These refined carbohydrates and simple sugars are quickly digested and converted into glucose, which rapidly enters the bloodstream and causes blood glucose levels to surge. Rapid swings in blood glucose levels produce excessive stress on the pancreas to secrete insulin and are unhealthy even for the "fit person." For the diabetic, whose disease is a lack of insulin, rapid swings cause real trouble. In very simple terms, refined diets loaded with sugars can "flog the pancreas" to dysfunction or death (the cessation of its ability to produce insulin).

In contrast, several studies have shown that complex carbohydrates—*i.e.*, whole grains, legumes (including soybeans), beans, and fresh vegetables and fruits, are digested more slowly and hence, glucose is absorbed into the bloodstream in a more even manner. For example, consuming a glass of apple juice, a simple carbohydrate, will cause a more rapid rise in blood sugar than eating a whole apple, a complex carbohydrate. Good diets do not gyrate the levels of glucose in the blood!

It was a major breakthrough for the treatment of diabetes when a connection was firmly established between a diet high in complex carbohydrates and a resulting management or even reversal of Type II diabetes. Today, many adult diabetic patients are able to avoid oral medication or insulin injections entirely if they plan their diets carefully and add an exercise program.

Much about the role of fiber and, therefore, the benefits of complex carbohydrates for dealing with diabetes was gleaned from examining societies in which diabetes is a rare or even nonexistent disease. For example, diabetes is virtually unknown in societies in which fiber intake is high and refined foods are rare. However, indigenous populations whose diets change as a result of urbanization and industrialization soon become vulnerable to diabetes—and a host of other conditions—because their changes in diet usually include greater quantities of refined foods.

SOYBEANS ARE OF SPECIAL VALUE IN DIABETES MELLITUS

Soybeans contain the types of soluble fiber that are valuable in slowing the release of glucose into the blood. The soluble fiber in soybeans has the ability to "smooth out" blood glucose levels, especially following meals. The gel that forms when soluble fiber combines with liquid is probably responsible for this slowing of the rate of absorption of glucose into the bloodstream. Other legumes, oats, barley, and fruit, such as apples, also contain this insulin-sparing type of soluble fiber.

My personal interest in soybeans was triggered by research I did on the effects of gel fibers (soluble types of fiber) on the absorption of blood glucose in humans. When I was a lecturer at the medical school at the University of Edinburgh, Scotland, my colleagues and I described the effects of gel fiber on the absorption of glucose in humans. This work, published in *Lancet* in 1979, showed that gel fibers, such as guar gum and pectin, delayed the rate at which the human stomach emptied its contents into the small bowel, which is the site of maximal absorption of glucose. Thus, gel fibers have the ability to reduce the rate at which glucose is absorbed and smooth out the levels of glucose achieved in the blood following their ingestion in the diet. Subsequent studies have confirmed these effects of gel fibers (soluble fibers) found in a variety of fruits, vegetables, and plants, including the mighty soybean.

A study of obese patients with Type II diabetes, published in the *American Journal of Clinical Nutrition* in 1987, showed the benefit of soy fiber in regulating blood glucose levels. The subjects were first given a meal that did not contain soy fiber, then their blood glucose levels were measured. As is typical in diabetic individuals, glucose levels rose rapidly and stayed high for longer than normal. However, when the same patients consumed an identical meal to which 10 grams of soy fiber were added, blood glucose levels returned to normal more quickly. Other studies have confirmed these findings. In one clinical experiment soy fiber and cellulose, an insoluble fiber found in bran and vegetables, were compared in relation to their effects on blood sugar. Those participants in the experiment given soy fiber had lower blood glucose levels over a three-hour period than the participants who received cellulose.

In addition, the fiber in soy food products helps promote a sense of fullness or satiety, which can be important for overweight diabetics, a group for whom weight loss is essential. Anyone who has tried to diet knows that a constant sense of hunger is detrimental and ultimately tends to lead to overeating, usually followed by another period during which too little food is consumed. A person with diabetes mellitus cannot safely engage in this "see-saw" of deprivation followed by overeating. Stabilizing the balance of glucose and insulin is impossible without careful planning and a disciplined approach to diet. Therefore, a food that promotes a sense of satiety is of supreme value in assisting weight loss where required.

The amino acid composition of soy protein helps explain some of the beneficial effects of soy food on glucose absorption. Soy protein contains large amounts of glycine and arginine, which tend to reduce blood insulin levels. Low blood insulin levels may act to decrease the synthesis of cholesterol in the liver. This is highly desirable in the diabetic individual, who is frequently affected by the consequences of hypercholesterolemia (high blood cholesterol). In contrast, animal proteins are low in these two amino acids, and contain more lysine than vegetable proteins as well. Lysine tends to raise insulin levels, and it promotes synthesis of cholesterol. A large proportion of medical practitioners and dieticians continue to recommend animal-protein based diets for diabetics or exercise permissiveness in their recommendations concerning them. At the same time, patients are instructed to consume fewer calories and cut their fat intake. A vegetable-protein based diet that emphasizes soy foods accomplishes this and directly acts to lower cholesterol, yet it is rarely promoted in medical practices. This simply does not make good sense to me.

SOY AND OTHER COMPLICATIONS OF DIABETES

Many diabetics must deal with a triad of problems—obesity, high cholesterol levels, and hypertension. The insoluble fiber that helps regulate blood glucose is the same type of fiber that helps lower blood cholesterol, making it a doubly desirable food for diabetics who are at high risk of developing heart disease. High fat levels in the blood is one of the complicating factors in managing diabetes, and atherosclerosis contributes to premature death in the diabetic population. Soy protein containing isoflavones have both preventive and therapeutic value for cardiovascular diseases, making it particularly valuable for diabetics.

Soy's ability to lower cholesterol, plus its lecithin content, are believed to be protective against gallstone formation, another condition that diabetics are prone to develop. In addition, people with diabetes may often develop specific digestive diseases. A condition called "diabetic diarrhea" is quite common, and this is probably most often related to damage of nerves that supply the gut (autonomic neuropathy). The content of soluble fiber in some soy foods can assist in regulating bowel habits that may be disturbed in individuals with long-standing diabetes. A high fiber diet, so beneficial for regulating blood sugar, is an effective way to prevent or manage an array of digestive diseases.

One of the most common—and devastating—complications of diabetes mellitus is diabetic retinopathy, a condition in which the capillaries in the eye increase in number (proliferate) and sometimes hemorrhage into the retina. In many cases of long-standing diabetes, new and fragile blood vessels grow on the surface of the retina. If these blood vessels bleed inside the eye, fibrous tissue can grow forward into the gel of the eyeball. It is possible that the isoflavones in soy, which have an antiangiogenic effect—meaning that they interfere with new blood vessel growth—could be of some value in controlling diabetic retinopathy. This use of soy isoflavones is worthy of more scientific investigation.

People with diabetes mellitus are at increased risk of kidney disorders, but they are often not told that soy protein is more easily handled by the kidneys than is animal protein. Yet, diabetes and/or hypertension (diabetics are at increased risk for developing high blood pressure) account for about half of the new kidney dialysis patients each year in the United States. According to recent studies, modest amounts of soy protein are able to lower diastolic blood pressure significantly and systolic blood pressure modestly. Nephrotic syndrome, a recognized complication of diabetes mellitus, is a serious disease that results when the filtering mechanisms of the kidneys are damaged. Clinical investigations have revealed that, while soy protein is handled by the kidneys more efficiently than animal protein, this is even more true when the comparison is made in the presence of the nephrotic syndrome. The administration of soy protein to individuals with nephrotic syndrome, replacing animal protein, has led to measurable improvements in kidney function.

In any patient, diabetic or not, who is demonstrating signs of kidney failure, it may be beneficial to avoid animal protein and switch to soy foods as the primary source of protein. Later chapters in this book will discuss the benefits of soy in both the prevention and treatment of a variety of conditions, many of which are associated with diabetes mellitus. While diabetes is a complex and potentially devastating condition, adequate self-care, along with insulin or oral medication when essential, enables many diabetics to live long, productive lives. Adding soy to the diet is a valuable addition to a self-care plan for any individual with diabetes mellitus. Equally important, however, is the role that soybeans and a vegetable-protein based diet may play in helping to prevent the disease in the first place.

DISABILITY AND DEATH IN DIABETES MELLITUS

It is a rotten thing that diabetes mellitus can compromise the quality of life experienced by at least 2 percent of the entire population of many Western countries, and that it causes premature death. The fact is, however, that the main medical complications of diabetes—cardiovascular disease and kidney impairment—are both amenable to variable correction by soy supplementation of the diet. Soy protein containing isoflavones lowers blood cholesterol in an unequivocal manner in many individuals, and similar soy foods may lower blood pressure. I stress that it is combination of *soy protein with isoflavones* that are needed to achieve the successful lowering of blood cholesterol.

By virtue of their protein composition, soy foods tend to be kind to the kidneys and they assist greatly in the management of kidney impairment in diabetes mellitus. Whether or not soy foods can prevent kidney damage in diabetes mellitus by improving the control of diabetes or perhaps by an antiangiogenic action on the diseased glomerulus remains to be studied. In the meantime, soy is being greatly underestimated as a powerful weapon in the fight against diabetes mellitus.

CHAPTER 7

Keeping Your Genito-Urinary Tract Healthy: Kidneys and Prostate

The kidneys have the important—and complex—function of being the body's filtering system: their job is to filter out undesirable chemicals from the blood and excrete them through the urine. Typically, the kidneys filter forty-five gallons of blood per day and, in the process, help to regulate the body's fluid balance.

The kidneys have numerous additional functions. They produce a hormone that regulates the formation of red blood cells in the bone marrow, and they convert vitamin D into a usable, active form. These special organs are also involved in regulating blood pressure, which is the reason why diminished kidney function is linked with hypertension. High blood pressure may be both a cause and a result of damage to the kidney.

Unfortunately, kidney function can be compromised by many conditions and disorders. Kidney infections are common; if left untreated, they can cause severe problems. In the nephrotic syndrome, a condition in which the kidneys are damaged, excessive amounts of protein are lost through the urine, which causes fluid to collect in tissues of the body (edema). Renal failure results when the kidneys' filtering system is severely impaired by blockage or damage, and chemical waste products accumulate in the blood and tissues.

Chronic kidney failure is a progressive condition, sometimes resulting from underlying conditions such as high blood pressure and diabetes mellitus. It is also a contributing factor in deaths caused by several degenerative diseases, such as cardiac disease and atherosclerosis, which are discussed elsewhere in this book. The treatment of significant renal disease is difficult, and the prevention of urinary tract diseases and maintenance of good renal function are very important for health. Soy fractions may have a special role to play in the prevention and treatment of kidney disease. After infections in the urinary tract, the most common condition affecting the kidneys—and potentially the entire urinary tract—is the presence of calculi, more commonly called stones.

KIDNEY STONE FORMATION

Formation of stones in the urinary tracts, particularly in the kidneys, is a very common condition in Western populations, but its prevalence is often underestimated. Nearly one person in a thousand will form a stone that may cause him or her to seek medical attention. While the majority of kidney and bladder stones occur in men, women must be aware of this condition, too. The pain caused by a stone may become excruciating and even frightening, often leading to a trip to the emergency room. On the other hand, some kidney stones, and those formed elsewhere in the urinary tract, are "silent," meaning that they do not produce symptoms or signs. However, these silent urinary stones can contribute to urinary infections and diminished kidney function because they cause blockages and stasis of urine, which is often accompanied by bacterial infection.

Every person should learn how urinary stones can be prevented, but for individuals who have a history of stone formation, it is of critical importance because this condition tends to recur. About 60 percent of individuals treated for a kidney stone will develop another one within seven years. Therefore, some individuals are prone to stone formation and are at higher risk throughout their lives. The likelihood of stone recurrence is very important because it means that preventive measures, often involving dietary adjustments, must be made in many individuals.

About 80 to 90 percent of urinary tract stones contain calcium; about 5 to 8 percent are composed of uric acid (a substance normally present in human urine in very small amounts); and approximately 2 percent contain cysteine, an amino acid in which sulphur is a notable component. It is likely that a large number of kidney stones are preventable by dietary adjustments, even among individuals who are prone to stone formation.

Dehydration is a common cause of kidney stones. One important preventive measure is to increase fluid intake in order to avoid low urine volumes. On average, individuals prone to forming stones should try to maintain fluid intake so that they excrete about three liters of urine per day. The general recommendation that everyone daily consume six to eight 8-ounce glasses of water is especially important for stone-forming persons or for others when they are at risk for dehydration. You can become dehydrated when you engage in strenuous physical activity or experience excessive sweating and do not replace the lost body fluid.

In addition, stone formation is often linked with elevated calcium or uric acid levels in the urine. The issue is, of course, what causes excessive calcium to be excreted. Diets high in animal protein promote excessive calcium loss through the urine. This cause-and-effect relationship between animal protein-based diets and calcium loss is also linked to the development of osteoporosis, a disease discussed in Chapter 10.

TOO MUCH ANIMAL PROTEIN

The typical Western diet, which includes large quantities of animal protein, can reasonably be considered a risk factor for developing kidney stones. Athletes who increase their consumption of animal protein as part of their conditioning are at risk of developing urinary tract stones because they sweat excessively; if they do not continually replace lost fluid, their urine becomes concentrated. This situation creates the ideal condition for stone formation.

It must be emphasized that there is a much higher incidence of kidney stones among populations favoring animal protein-based diets than among those whose staple diet is vegetable-based. In an American study of 450,000 men, those whose diets were highest in animal protein were at far greater risk for producing a kidney stone containing calcium than men whose diets contained more moderate amounts of animal protein. A British study showed a greatly reduced risk of developing kidney stones among vegetarians. Throughout the world, those who consume soy-based diets tend to have a relatively low incidence of kidney stones.

REDUCING CALCIUM INTAKE IS NOT NECESSARILY WISE

In the West, where the advantages of vegetarian diets are less well-known and accepted, the medical community is still debating the optimal ways to prevent kidney stones. Some nutritionists and physicians recommend restricting calcium, which appears to be a logical recommendation—if one does not consider the body's need for calcium. However, no controlled studies have demonstrated a clear reduction in urinary stone formation as a result of restricting calcium intake. In fact, an important study reported in the *New England Journal of Medicine* showed the reverse effect. In other words, increasing calcium in the diet actually led to a reduction in the incidence of stone formation. Individuals with the highest calcium intake showed a 50 percent reduction in kidney stones when compared to those with the lowest intake. There are a few isolated circumstances in which decreasing calcium may be beneficial in patients with renal disease, but for the majority of individuals it is often not necessary. The matter of dietary intake of calcium and vitamin D in individuals with kidney disease is complex, and the advice of a medical practitioner should always be sought in cases of doubt.

THE TYPE OF PROTEIN CONSUMED IS THE KEY

There is considerable evidence that vegetable protein, particularly soy protein, is more efficiently handled by the kidneys than animal protein. For example, one study demonstrated that patients with nephrotic syndrome benefited from dietary treatment that included soy protein. Nephrotic syndrome is a kidney disease that results in protein loss in the urine, edema (fluid retention) in variable degrees, and high levels of lipids (fats) in the blood. Several studies have found that protein loss through the urine was decreased when soy protein replaced animal protein in subjects with renal disease. Blood cholesterol levels also decreased in patients with renal failure who were given soy protein. These beneficial results on normalizing blood fats (cholesterol) is similar to the results of other research that has shown the cholesterol lowering-effects of soy. Hypertension (high blood pressure) is invariably associated with renal failure and, as we learned earlier, soy protein seems to exert an antihypertensive effect.

Protein loss through the urine is higher when the kidneys are not working efficiently, and that has led some clinicians to recommend reducing the amount of total protein consumed, a treatment that presents problems of its own. It appears, though, that the important factor is not the amount but the type of protein consumed. Again, because soy protein is efficiently handled by the kidneys, those with reduced kidney function will benefit from a vegetable-protein based diet that emphasizes soy. Remember that soy is a complete protein, and therefore is an adequate substitute for meat, poultry, fish, and dairy products.

SOY FOR THE ELDERLY KIDNEY

Because the kidneys become less efficient as we age, soy is an ideal source of protein for the elderly. If we look at the incidence of diseases that contribute to kidney failure, particularly hypertension, cardiovascular conditions, and diabetes mellitus, then we can see that these are the very diseases that afflict so many elderly people. Among the younger population, these diseases make people "old" before their time in that they adversely affect "quality of life," regardless of age.

Currently, moderately restricting protein and regulating calcium and phosphorus intake is a treatment for kidney failure that is accepted by many experts in the field. Kidney failure is generally a progressive disease, and the goal of this treatment is to retard its progression. One of the consequences of kidney failure is uremia—that is, high levels of urea in the blood. (Urea is a major waste product of protein metabolism; excessive build-up of urea is called uremia, a condition associated with multiple problems.) Since many patients with kidney failure lose excessive protein in the urine, it is necessary to then add protein to compensate for the loss. Given these circumstances, soy protein should be considered because it is well tolerated in the diet and appears to be far more easily "handled" by the kidneys than animal protein. In other words, if kidney function is already compromised, then treatment should lessen the stress on these organs rather than add to their burden. In simple terms, animal protein appears to force the kidneys to work harder, so restricting its intake is beneficial.

As you can see, soy protein has the potential to help prevent kidney stones and other chronic kidney diseases. Undoubtedly, dietary recommendations for persons who suffer from disorders of the kidneys are complex and require medical supervision. I am not suggesting that you ignore medical advice; however, I am suggesting that many medical practitioners are unaware of the benefits of soy. In a conventional practitioner's office, you will likely be offered treatments based on their current popularity in the medical community rather than on new information about the benefits and safety of soy.

Because soy food products have numerous advantages, it makes sense to incorporate them into your diet to improve the underlying conditions that have caused chronic kidney failure. In other words, using soy protein may be considered as both a life-long preventive measure and a treatment for existing problems affecting the urinary tract. Please talk with your doctor about this.

THE MENOPAUSAL URINARY TRACT

Stress incontinence (weak bladder), recurrent urinary tract infections, vaginal dryness, and atrophy of the vulva are troublesome consequences of the menopause. Menopause is discussed in detail in Chapter 9, but it is worth noting that there are many anecdotal reports of improvements of genito-urinary function in menopausal females given soy supplements. Soy isoflavones seem to be especially beneficial in reversing the vaginal dryness that so often interferes with sexual intercourse in mature couples.

SPECIAL CONCERNS FOR MEN

The prostate gland produces secretions that are part of the seminal fluid and other secretions that keep the lining of the urethra moist. The gland is small at birth, but begins to enlarge when the production of androgen increases during puberty and adolescence. By age twenty or so, the prostate gland weighs about 20 grams and stays stable until around age fifty, when it often begins to enlarge. Though its cause often is not known completely, this enlargement is so common that it is considered an expected part of aging—hence the term, benign prostatic enlargement. (The prostate also enlarges in the presence of cancer, in which case it is referred to as malignant prostatic enlargement. It has been stated that the chance of developing prostate cancer is 90 percent in a male who reaches the age of ninety years.)

For many men prostatic enlargement is a slow process and presents little or no difficulty throughout their lives. Despite having the term "benign" applied to it, enlargement of the prostate is not always a benign condition because it very frequently causes obstruction of the urinary tract. The enlarging prostate can compress the urethra, resulting in a weaker urinary stream, "dribbling" urine, and sometimes difficulty with initiating urination.

Sometimes the symptoms of benign prostatic enlargement become serious enough that a surgical removal of the prostate gland is recommended. Unfortunately, prostate surgery commonly causes sexual dysfunction, such as delayed or absent ejaculation, and it may even cause incontinence in some individuals. Because surgery is an extreme step, nonsurgical treatment is favored when possible. Currently, hormonal drug therapy is receiving wide attention as a less drastic but potentially effective treatment.

ANDROGEN, ESTROGEN, AND THE PROSTATE GLAND

Although the exact causes of benign or malignant prostatic disease remain unknown, virtually all accounts of the subject stress the importance of hormonal factors in their development. The common theory of the development of benign prostatic hyperplasia (BPH) includes a role for prostatic build-up of dihydrotestosterone (DHT), a hormone that promotes prostatic growth. Many therapies for prostatic disease focus on the reduction of DHT levels, primarily by interfering with 5-alpha-reductase.

In any case hormone therapy for prostate enlargement is aimed at modulating the effects of both the male hormone androgen and female estrogen. Hormonal therapy is effective, in that the enlargement is reversed when the prostate is deprived of the stimulating effects of androgen. Finasteride, the generic name for Proscar, is a widely used drug for prostatic hyperplasia, or excessive proliferation of cells in the prostate gland. The drug produces a fall in the serum and prostate gland levels of a specific androgenic hormone (dihydrotestosterone). It is claimed that 30 percent of patients who use the drug for six months will have about a 30 percent reduction in the size of the prostate. However, since prostate enlargement recurs when the drug is stopped, treatment with it has to be long-term. As a result some clinicians have concluded that finasteride should be used as a life-long therapy. In the short term the drug is probably safe; however, the long-term effects remain unknown, and there is no scientific reason to conclude that the drug is safe for life-long use.

Along with other practitioners of alternative medicine, Dr. Michael Schachter, past president of two leading medical societies, has expressed his opinion that finasteride may cause prostate cancer in the long-term. Dr. Schachter's book, *Good Health Guide, The Natural Way to a Healthy Prostate*, includes a complete discussion of the causes of diseases of the prostate. He also includes many lifestyle, nutritional, and dietary recommendations that readers may find useful. I highly recommend Dr. Schachter's informative book.

The tremendous potential value of the weak estrogens, isoflavones, present in soy protein isolates for both the prevention and treatment of benign prostatic enlargement has been staring the medical profession in the face for some time now. Nonetheless, its efficacy is still all but ignored by conventional practitioners. Add to this the pervasive unwillingness among members of the medical community to accept that dietary factors can contribute anything at all to the treatment of both benign and malignant prostatic disease, and we are left with the dismal prospect that millions of men will be offered synthetic pharmaceuticals for their problems. Yet isoflavones appear to be able to act to modulate the harmful effects of hormones in benign prostatic enlargement. Nature seems to have "manufactured" an option for mature men in the form of soy isoflavones, adaptogens, which modulate hormonal (estrogenic) activity in the body.

ISOFLAVONES AND PROSTATIC DISEASE

Demographic studies have drawn attention to the lower incidence of prostatic disease among Japanese men compared with Western men, especially older men. At least in part, this difference can be attributed to the influence of a soy-based diet in Japanese men. The soy isoflavones genistein and daidzein appear to directly affect testosterone metabolism and reduce the formation of toxic types of testosterone. Clearly, more research is needed to define the role of soy in maintaining a healthy prostate gland. However, what we already know about the benefits of isoflavones is currently leading many alternative or integrative health practitioners to recommend using soy and isolated soy isoflavones therapeutically, to prevent and treat benign enlargement of the prostate.

In an excellent study of the demographics and diet of men of Japanese ancestry living in Hawaii, it was found that the incidence of prostate cancer was substantially less in those individuals consuming soy in their diet. This study was important because it was a prospective study performed over a twenty-year period. Of the 8,000 men studied, it was found that those who consumed tofu once a week or less were three times more likely to get prostate cancer than those who ate tofu daily. Tofu was found to be the most protective form of soy food in the study, and it is rich in both protein and isoflavones.

The hormonal modulating effects of isoflavones are likely the key to their preventing benign prostate enlargement because estrogens play a role in causing prostate problems. This issue certainly warrants further investigation because soy isoflavones do not present the problems with side effects associated with potent estrogens or other synthetically produced antiandrogenic substances.

The theory that isoflavones, with their weak estrogenic effects, is beneficial for prostatic disease is akin to the theory that the effect of weak estrogens may help prevent breast cancer. When isoflavones occupy the receptor sites in the prostate, the effects of more dangerously potent natural—or synthetic—estrogens are blocked, just as they are in the breast.

It appears that isoflavones may have a significant role in preventing the prostatic diseases that are rampant in mature males. Obviously, further scientific validation of the protective role of isoflavones against prostatic disease is necessary. However, this theory goes a long way in explaining the lower incidence of hormonally dependent cancers among populations such as the

Japanese, for whom soy is a dietary staple. It is also significant that when the diets of Asians become more Westernized and include fewer soy foods, rates for these cancers rise.

Dr. Herman Adlercreutz, professor in the Department of Clinical Chemistry at the University of Helsinki, has performed a great deal of research on the effects of soy fractions—in particular, soy isoflavones—on the maintenance of prostate health. Laboratory experiments with cultures of prostate cancer cells show an antitumor effect of soy isoflavones, and several animal studies have shown that transplanted prostate cancer in animals can have its growth retarded by genistein (a principal soy isoflavone).

Current research and clinical experience is leading more and more health care practitioners to recommend that mature men add at least two servings of soy food products to their daily diets. In addition, isoflavone supplements are available to both prevent and treat benign prostatic enlargement and possibly cancer of the prostate. I can provide many anecdotes from my own experiences with patients, including reports of beneficial effects of high isoflavone intake in advanced prostate cancer, and reversal of symptoms of benign prostatic hyperplasia with just modest intake of soy isoflavones. So important is the role of isoflavones in preventing prostatic disorders that Dr. Adlercreutz believes that every male should ingest soy isoflavones every day!

I caution that high doses of isoflavones should not be used without the supervision and advice of a health-care professional. In general, up to 80 mg of total isoflavones appear to be quite safe in the normal adult, but optimal doses are not known.

CHAPTER 8

Soy and Digestive Problems

Walk the aisles of any supermarket, and you can be impressed by the vast array of over-the-counter remedies for digestive upsets. When we consider the number of prescription and over-the-counter medications designed to "aid" digestion, it would appear that, like periodic headaches, digestive difficulties are nearly universal. This is a misguided belief. The good news is that many types of digestive upsets are preventable and can be safely treated when they do occur. Many natural remedies have been developed for settling an upset stomach or cranky bowel. Fiber is perhaps the most important of these natural remedies.

THE FIBER STORY

Dietary fiber comes from the supporting structure of plant foods and generally resists digestion in the human gastrointestinal tract. Although there are many types of fiber, they are generally described as belonging to either of two broad categories: soluble and insoluble. Soluble fiber tends to disperse in water and form a gel, but it is not absorbed into the bloodstream. Insoluble fiber also holds water (is hydroscopic), but it travels through the digestive tract virtually intact. Soybeans and legumes in general contain significant amounts of soluble fiber. The husks of soy-beans contain an insoluble fiber called lignin as well.

In 1980 two scientists, Neil Painter, M.D., and Denis Burkitt, M.D., proposed that a lack of adequate fiber in the diet may be a key factor in predisposing many individuals to some of the common chronic diseases that afflict Western societies. They found that societies in which fiber intake was high—that is, societies that were largely vegetarian—had a much lower incidence of several chronic diseases, including colon cancer, heart disease, and most digestive disorders, than in Western societies.

The change in diet—and resulting rise in certain diseases—among mobile populations also added credibility to Painter and Burkitt's fiber hypothesis. For example, Japanese people born in Hawaii have diverticular disease and colon cancer with a frequency similar to that of white Americans, while Japanese people living in Japan have a relatively low incidence of these colonic diseases.

Once it was recognized that fiber had a therapeutic role in preventing and treating many digestive disorders, the work of Burkitt and Painter became a "hot" topic in the West. From high-fiber cereals to wheat bran supplements to oat bran muffins and simple advice to add more fresh fruits and vegetables to the diet, fiber quickly became a focus of both the medical and the lay communities.

Many people think of bran as the most valuable source of fiber, primarily because it has been superbly marketed to "promote regularity" of the bowels. In fact, insoluble fibers are sometimes referred to as bulk laxatives. However, the soluble fibers found in soybeans also regulate bowel action. They are fermented in the colon to produce short-chain fatty acids, which stimulate colonic activity, but the insoluble fiber found in soy does not make the stool too bulky.

Adding Fiber Every Day

Most people consuming a Western diet have a deficient intake of fiber, often amounting to less than 10 grams of fiber per day. Vegetarians may eat an average of 40 grams of fiber per day versus 20 to 25 grams a day for those eating the "recommended"

Western diet. If we consider only the benefits of fiber for digestive health, it is not surprising that vegetarians have far fewer digestive complaints. Existing research suggests that increasing fiber intake can relieve or assist in control of the symptoms of diverticulosis and some cases of functional bowel disease and inflammatory bowel disease. Equally important, adequate fiber has been shown to reduce blood cholesterol, and the soluble type of fiber found in soybeans is particularly up to this task. (See Chapter 4.)

It is ironic that, until fairly recently, individuals with gastrointestinal complaints were often advised to reduce their fiber intake. Some people believe that they must reduce fiber as they age because their systems can no longer "handle" whole grains and raw foods. However, reducing fiber often exacerbates several symptoms, such as the stubborn bowels and abdominal aches that commonly affect mature individuals. Recommendations within the medical community have changed as data confirming the value of including fiber in the diet accumulate.

Be Wise: Add Fiber Slowly

A common mistake among individuals who "get religion," so to speak, about fiber, is to increase dietary fiber intake too quickly. Some abdominal bloating and excessive gas formation are inevitable during an initial period of adjustment to added fiber in the diet. For this reason, it is best to add fiber to the diet gradually over a period of weeks, rather than try to increase intake to the optimal amount within a day or two. It is best to work through the transient unpleasantness that commonly occurs in the early stages of the healthful inclusion of fiber in the diet.

Vegetarians have little difficulty consuming adequate fiber in their diet because the variety of grains, beans, legumes, fruits, and vegetables in their diet tend to provide good, balanced mixtures of soluble and insoluble fiber. Because it contains both soluble and insoluble fibers, soy is an ideal source of fiber, especially when taken in a traditional Asian formats. Unfortunately, the "refining" of soybeans to match the appeal of the Western palate has led to many commercially available soy foods that are deficient in soy fiber.

SOY AND A HEALTHY COLON

The soluble fiber in soy may have a specific role in preventing colon cancer. This is a complex issue that involves the production and balance of bacteria in the colon. High protein intake may result in the production of nitrosamines by bacteria. Nitrosamines are known to promote tumor growth. The harmful effects of nitrosamines on the cells of the lining of the colon can be limited by the presence of short-chain fatty acids produced by the activity of bacteria on dietary fiber, such as the soluble fiber and complex carbohydrates found in soybeans. Short-chain fatty acids promote a beneficial environment in the colon, which helps to interfere with the potential cancer-promoting actions of nitrosamines.

In addition, this "friendly" environment alters the metabolism of the body's own bile acids that reach the colon so that these bile acids are not changed into potential carcinogens. By promoting this "friendly" bacterial environment, soy fiber can exert a potentially protective effect against colon cancer and other gastrointestinal diseases.

Soy also can be important for promoting the growth of favorable bacteria in the colon. The way this comes about is through the operation of several types of complex sugars present in soybeans. These sugars are oligosaccharides (complicated types of nondigestible carbohydrates that enter the colon), such as raffinose and stachyose. These oligosaccharides provide a principal source of energy for bacterial growth in the form of fermentable carbohydrates. Certain "friendly" bacteria in the colon may metabolize oligosaccharides and thrive and grow. These friendly types of bacteria may metabolize (get rid of) carcinogens. The destruction of carcinogenic compounds by friendly bacteria is a protective effect that can be indirectly attributed to the occurrence of nondigestible carbohydrates (oligosaccharides) in soy-based diets.

An example of a friendly bacterium that benefits from soy-based diets is bifidobacteria, which is known to cause a reduced amount of carcinogenic compounds in the stool. Studies conducted in Japan have also shown a relationship between bifidobacteria in the colon and longevity. For example, one study focused on elderly Japanese individuals, some of whom lived in rural areas while others lived in urban settings. The rural dwellers relied on soybeans as a staple food to a greater extent than their urban counterparts. Researchers found that those in rural areas had greater amounts of bifidobacteria in their colons than those living in urban areas. The rural people had greater life expectancy than the urban dwellers. While it is not possible to establish an absolute cause-and-effect relationship, the results of the study are intriguing, particularly since oligosaccharides have been revered by many Japanese people as a "longevity" aid. The idea that indigestible, complex carbohydrates such as raffinose and stachyose can promote longevity has produced a great demand for certain types of soy flour containing these carbohydrates, which are used in Japan as dietary supplements.

HOW MUCH FIBER DO YOU NEED?

There is agreement about fiber intake among several major health organizations, including the American Diabetes Association and the National Cancer Institute, both of whom set their recommendations at 20 to 35 grams a day. The Reference Daily Intake (RDI) of dietary fiber proposed by the FDA for labeling purposes on nutritional products in the United States is 25 grams a day. This recommendation matches those of several European countries and those made by the Department of Health in Australia.

The World Health Organization (WHO) has been more specific in defining dietary fiber requirements by expressing recommendations in terms of nonstarch polysaccharides. Expressed this way, their recommendation for nonstarch polysaccharides is 16 to 24 grams a day, which is consistent with estimates of 27 to 40 grams of total dietary fiber a day.

THE SPECIAL VALUE OF SOY FIBERS

The best way to measure the value of any fiber is by demonstrating its clinical effects. In this regard, the benefits of both soluble and insoluble soy fiber derived from whole soybeans have been shown in many studies. For example, soy fiber has been shown to play a significant role in normalizing bowel function, controlling both constipation and diarrhea. "Transit time" through the gastrointestinal tract is also favorably altered when soy is consumed. Even small additions of soy fiber can bring beneficial results.

Since it reduces cholesterol, as well as promotes regular bowel function, soy fiber is, in my opinion, superior to psyllium hydrophilic mucilloid, better known by the brand name Metamucil. In another health area, a study has shown that soy fiber is beneficial in controlling diarrhea in infants, without demonstrating negative effects on nutrient absorption or nutritional status.

Common digestive diseases are largely preventable by consuming a diet that includes at least the minimum fiber recommendations endorsed by private health organizations and governmental agencies. Fiber is also part of the treatment for these conditions once they begin. For average consumers, there appears to be a clear choice—rely on myriad medications to relieve symptoms, or gradually make changes in diet by adding fiber from a variety of sources, including soy, and avoid gastointestinal diseases in the first place.

More Advantages of Soy

Many health-care professionals and patients are concerned about adding fiber to the diet because it has been shown to interfere with the absorption of certain minerals. A major advantage of soy fiber over several other types of dietary fiber, including bran, is that it does not tend to substantially affect mineral absorption. Wheat bran has been shown to lower zinc and copper absorption, but soy fiber does not exert this effect to the same degree.

I am not saying that soy fiber should necessarily be your primary source of fiber, or that you have to avoid wheat and oat bran. Balancing the sources and types of fiber in your diet is probably the best plan. However, when you are considering the sources of total dietary fiber, soy should be one of your choices. Given its known ability to lower cholesterol, protect against gallstone formation, and help regulate blood sugar, as well as its potential to protect against several forms of cancer, traditional soy food diets are too valuable to ignore. Protecting against digestive diseases is one advantage of soy fiber among many.

If you are currently suffering from a digestive disorder, ask your health-care provider to work with you on improving your condition with diet. While adding soy foods to your diet is almost always safe, I do not recommend that you add large amounts of fiber without first seeking advice from a qualified health-care giver.

CHAPTER 9

Omnipause: Both Sexes Should Read This

I have coined the term "omnipause" because the "pause of life" is not an event unique to females. There is increasing recognition of the male equivalent of the menopause, a time of life that has been termed the "andropause." Changes for both the female menopause and the male andropause occur over a varying time span. The term "climacteric" may better describe the protracted changes that occur in both women and men. However, because the changes are so different for each sex, menopause and andropause must be discussed separately.

THE MENOPAUSE

I recognize that many women object to having stages in their lives defined solely in reproductive terms. First they enter puberty, followed by several decades often defined as the reproductive years, and then, along comes menopause and the post-reproductive, or postmenopausal years. Even more objectionable to many women are the terms "the change," or "the change of life." As physician Susan Love says in *Dr. Susan Love's Hormone Book: Making Informed Choices about Menopause*: "Menopause is a change. Not 'the' change, but 'a' change. . . ."

Just as puberty is a transition from childhood into adolescence, and the capacity to bear children, menopause is a transition to mid-life, when a woman stops ovulating and menstruation ceases. In Western societies, about one in five or six women go through the menopause without major discomfort, whereas approximately the same number have quite severe symptoms and require intensive supportive care. The remainder have variable discomfort of moderate severity.

What to Expect

To attempt to describe an average woman's experience with menopause is nearly impossible, but there are broad descriptions. The perimenopause usually lasts two to five years and starts when a woman is between ages forty-five to fifty-five. Some women begin experiencing symptoms in their early forties, and surgical removal of the uterus and ovaries will trigger a premature menopause, regardless of age. While there is a group of common symptoms, their duration or intensity is individual, and about 10 percent of women never experience them at all. These women simply stop having periods, and that is the only way they know they have passed through menopause.

Although the list of symptoms associated with menopause is long, some occur frequently enough to be considered typical. These include:

- hot flashes
- night sweats
- sleep disturbances (some of which are linked with night sweats)
- vaginal dryness
- headaches
- heavy, light, or irregular menstrual flow
- frequent urination and cystitis
- mood swings
- fluctuations in libido
- pain in the lower back and other muscle and joint discomfort
- digestive difficulties

Other symptoms include depression, periodic sensitivity to touch, a tendency to gain weight on the upper body, bouts with anxiety or occasional panic attacks, an inability to concentrate, and memory lapses. Any one of these symptoms sounds annoying at the very least, and taken together, it is easy to understand why some women approach this time of life with a sense of dread.

Hormone Replacement Therapy

In earlier discussions, we considered estrogen and its effects on women. These matters are of great importance in relationship to soy and will be reiterated. When a woman stops ovulating, her ovaries largely stop producing the hormones estrogen and progesterone. Hormone replacement therapy, or HRT, is supposed to restore a woman's hormonal balance, largely her estrogen level, to something closer to what it was in her premenopausal state. This sounds good in theory, and, for many women, it often eases menopausal symptoms and sometimes restores a sense of well-being. However, despite the way HRT is currently promoted, it may not be a "miracle" therapy, primarily because it brings with it problems of its own. In fact, only 30 percent of women ever fill a prescription for hormonal therapy they are given, probably because they are afraid. Other women start the therapy but stop on their own, and currently about 85 percent of postmenopausal women are not using HRT. Many women do not like the side-effects, or they fear the long-term risks.

Some physicians promote HRT as a "panacea" for problems other than menopausal symptoms. They point out that correcting estrogen imbalances is preventive for such chronic diseases as osteoporosis and heart disease that otherwise affect women in the postmenopausal years. As a result even those women who experience few if any menopausal symptoms take hormones in order to reduce their risk of developing these diseases later in life. HRT is also touted as the proverbial fountain of youth for women, which adds to its seductive appeal in our "youth-oriented" culture.

Indeed the promoters of HRT have, for several decades, created a dismal picture of the "untreated postmenopausal woman." The image is one of a woman plagued by depression, with dry and wrinkled skin, brittle bones, a sense that she has lost her sex appeal, and a host of other unflattering implications. This picture is a far cry from the one painted by anthropologist Margaret Mead when she coined the phrase "postmenopausal zest" to describe the positive feelings many women experience when they discover familiar concerns about childbearing and chil-drearing replaced by a new world of opportunities.

Is Medical Intervention Absolutely Necessary?

Though currently in a minority, some physicians still maintain a conservative approach to menopause. They believe that some symptoms are inevitable for most women and, because meno-pause is a natural process, no medical intervention is necessary. Rather than offer anyone this "suffer in silence" advice, I prefer to address the problems. If your personal and professional life is being adversely affected by the symptoms, you are not likely to think of them as small. It is probably not too much to say that the decision to use hormone replacement therapy or not is the single most difficult and important health-related decision a woman will make during her adult life.

If you do go with HRT, the disadvantages include increased risk of uterine cancer, an uncertain risk of breast cancer (meaning that existing studies appear to offer contradictory results), plus a higher risk of developing gall bladder disease and vascular thrombosis (blood clot). HRT almost always causes weight gain. Some side-effects include breakthrough bleeding, depression, and symptoms similar to those described for premenstrual syndrome, including dizziness, increased body and facial hair, and changes in libido. If you think this is beginning to sound like some of the symptoms of meno-pause itself, you are correct. In fact, one reason women say they stop taking HRT is that the "cure is worse than the disease."

To Take HRT or Suffer in Silence

Unfortunately women have been led to believe that they have only two alternatives: to take the potent estrogens of HRT (with or without progesterone), or not take them—and *both* alternatives are burdened with risk. The notion that HRT is the solution to menopause, and, moreover, that not taking it means that a woman must "suffer in silence," are two of the biggest misconceptions about menopause in modern medicine. Credible scientific research and even simple observation indicate that there are more choices than this for women facing menopause.

For example, many Asian women consuming soy diets do not seem to be as bothered by the symptoms of menopause as women in Western societies. Furthermore, the chronic degenerative diseases associated with the post-menopausal status do not appear to be quite so common in Asian females either. One survey of Japanese women noted that a specific word for "hot flash" does not exist in the Japanese language, and less than ten percent of women reported experiencing them. In fact, the most common symptom was "stiff shoulders," reported by 52 percent of the women surveyed. Other cross-cultural research confirms that in many societies menopause is not considered a medical issue and, in fact, is viewed as a positive transition.

At this point, the differences in diet appear to be the best explanation for the cultural differences in response to menopause. When Asian women move to the West and begin eating larger quantities of animal protein at the expense of vegetable and soy protein, they often experience the same array of menopausal symptoms as Western women. In many Asian countries, the diet not only tends to be vegetarian, although seldom exclusively so, but it also tends to emphasize various soy products. Tofu, tempeh, soy milk, steamed fresh soybeans, and soy flour are mainstays of the diet. As we learn more about soy and the health status of populations that eat large quantities of soy foods, it makes sense to investigate whether soy might hold the key to safely easing menopausal symptoms. I believe strongly that soy isoflavones are a viable alternative to HRT for menopausal females, and I have received pressure from some quarters for holding this viewpoint.

Phytoestrogens Enter the Picture

As I have explained elsewhere in this book, soybeans contain isoflavones, which are natural "weak" estrogens found in some plants—hence, the term "phytoestrogens." These isoflavones may represent the best alternative to hormone replacement therapy discovered to date. We know that isoflavones play an important role in cancer prevention and in preventing and treating cardio-vascular conditions and osteoporosis. (These diseases are dis-cussed in detail in Chapter 4 and Chapter 10, respectively.) What these benefits mean for postmenopausal women is that hormone replacement therapy may not be the only way to prevent degen-erative diseases as HRT alleviates some of the symptoms of menopause. In addition, phytoestrogens and soy protein are safe substances; at recommended levels of intake they present no known risks, and this lack of side effects makes them a superior alternative to synthetic and animal estrogens.

It is important to understand that the body itself produces estrogens of various potencies. When we use the word "estrogen," we are actually talking about three important forms of the female hormone: estrone (E1), estradiol (E2), and estriol (E3). Each has its own function. For example, estriol, along with progesterone, dominate during pregnancy. In simplistic terms, estrogens are responsible for "femininity," and they promote secondary sex characteristics in women. It should also be recognized that estro-gen is a powerful trophic, a word taken from the Greek word *trophikos*, meaning, in this context, growth. Estrogen is a hormone that stimulates all growth, but especially the growth of ductal tissues in the breast. The ability of estrogens to stimulate cell divi-sion, particularly in tissue that is sensitive to hormones, such as that in the breast and the lining of the uterus, is very important in understanding the possible carcinogenic effects of estrogen.

Of the three major types of estrogen, estradiol is the most stimulating to the breast tissue, while estriol has the weakest effect. Estradiol dominates in the formulas for the synthetic estrogens used in contraceptives and estrogen-replacement therapies, and it is probably responsible for some of the unpleasant side effects associated with both of them—and, of course, the increased risk of developing hormone-dependent cancers. On the other hand, the weaker estriol is theoretically the safer estrogen and is associated with effective treatment of vaginal dryness. The concept of two different strengths of estrogens, potent or weak, is important in gaining an understanding of the type of estrogens used in the pharmaceutical products marketed for menopause—and beyond.

The Benefits of Weak Estrogens

Plant estrogens serve a two-fold purpose in that they are both a source of estrogen-like compounds and have the ability to block the more potent estrogens. Thus, isoflavones can be considered "modulators" of estrogenic effects on tissues in the body. Some menopausal symptoms, such as hot flashes and vaginal dryness, are linked to reduced levels of estrogen; plant estrogens may serve to mimic estrogen and, therefore, prevent these unpleasant symptoms. In other words, soy isoflavones exert estrogenic effects in the absence of estrogen. On the other hand, plant estrogens can block the more powerful and potentially harmful effects that occur when abundant estrogens are produced by the body.

This is as good as it sounds. In situations where estrogen is lacking, isoflavones are estrogenic, whereas in situations where estrogen dominates, isoflavones are antiestrogenic. Thus isoflavones modulate the action of estrogen, and they can be proestrogenic or antiestrogenic, depending on the circumstances of prevailing estrogen dominance. Soy isoflavones have been described as ideal "adaptogens" (compounds that balance functions in the body) by several leading physicians and scientists.

Recently, reports about the benefits of the phytoestrogens in soy (isoflavones) to promote menopausal wellness have reached the popular press. This is a very positive development. Unfortunately, consumers are often given incomplete information. For example, several television reports have claimed that soy products, particularly tofu, can relieve hot flashes in menopausal women. What was not made clear is that eating tofu now and then will not provide the amount of isoflavones needed to produce the desired benefits. In fact, women who are experiencing regular hot flashes would have to eat a half pound of tofu—or more—*every day* to get sufficient isoflavones to have a positive effect, and even that amount does not guarantee a sufficient dose!

However, isoflavones in soy can be isolated and formulated into a dietary supplement designed to suppress menopausal symptoms and promote post-menopasual well-being. This is the kind of simple and practical information women need, and such supplements are gaining increasing popularity (such as Phyto-Est, manufactured by Biotherapies, Inc., Fairfield, New Jersey, and isoflavones sold by Nature's Way of Springville, Utah).

VARIATIONS IN ISOFLAVONE CONTENT OF SOY FOODS

The exact isoflavone content of any commercially available soy food cannot be reliable. As the growing conditions for soybeans and the nutrient content of soil vary, so the nutrient content of any soy-based food will also vary. Processing methods also influence the chemical composition of the end product. However, when a nutrient is isolated and designed to be used therapeutically, it then becomes a nutriceutical and production has to be designed to meet specific standards. Remember that the concept behind the use of nutriceuticals is not new. When patients with cardiovascular disease are instructed to take vitamin E, the nutrient is being used therapeutically and, at that point, it becomes a nutriceutical, not just a dietary supplement. However, I want to stress that you should not use on your own any dietary supplements for prevention or treatment of disease. I advise you to seek the guidance of a qualified health-care practitioner if you wish to use nutrients, botanicals, or herbs as medicines.

Therapeutic Value of Isoflavones

Soybeans contain two principal isoflavones, genistein and daidzein, and one minor one, glycitein. Their chemical composition includes a ring structure that resembles natural estrogens. Isoflavones appear to modulate (balance) estrogenic activity in the body in a consistent manner, which is what is meant when claims are made that isoflavones both provide estrogen to the body and block its potentially harmful effects. Isoflavones have the ability to bind to estrogen receptor sites in cells and prevent the more potent estrogens from affecting those cells.

Logical questions arise when discussing a nutriceutical. First, how do we know such a supplement is effective? And even if it is effective, is it safe? Is it relatively easy to use and affordable? The answers for isoflavones are in the research results, and they confirm that isoflavone supplementation is effective. The soy-based diet of Japanese women, for example, combined with their relative lack of troublesome menopausal symptoms, provide a model upon which to base the dosages used for research.

Using Isoflavones for Menopause Is Backed by Science

Prior to controlled studies, there was considerable anecdotal evidence that soy products were effective in relieving menopausal symptoms. Now, clinical studies in several countries have substantiated the anecdotal evidence. In one study, conducted by Dr. John Eden and his colleagues at the Royal Hospital for Women in New South Wales, Australia, participants were given 160 mg of soy isoflavones for three months. Several menopausal symptoms improved to a statistically significant degree, especially hot flashes.

Another study, performed at Tufts University School of Medicine in Boston, Massachusetts, resulted in a small decrease in menopausal symptoms, when compared to the women taking a placebo. Even a small decrease is significant because the isoflavone dosage was only 40 mg per day, as compared to the 160 mg used in the Australian study.

The results of a double-blind, crossover study conducted in Manchester, in the United Kingdom, are especially important because serum levels of growth hormone and two hormones involved in regulating the menstrual cycle—prolactin and luteinizing hormone—were higher when the participants were taking 80 mg of isoflavones per day. Blood cholesterol decreased as well. When the women took the placebo, the benefits disappeared. In addition, the women reported significant reduction of menopausal symptoms, particularly hot flashes, when on the isoflavone treatment, but not when they were taking the placebo. This study suggests that the estrogenic properties of isoflavones can act on the pituitary gland, which stimulates production of growth hormone and prolactin.

In a study conducted at Wake Forest University in North Carolina, Dr. Gregory Burke reported that soy isoflavones given to women in menopause alleviated the severity of their symptoms but did not duplicate the undesirable effects that were produced when the women were given synthetic or animal estrogens. Some women on pharmaceutical HRT show a rise in blood triglycerides and, in addition, increased cell growth in the breast and the endometrium (the lining of the uterus). These side effects are not minor, in that they account for the known increased risk of uterine and breast cancer from taking HRT. There is also an increased risk of blood clotting among women on HRT, while no such risk exists with isoflavone therapy. Dr. Burke was so impressed with the results from this test of using soy isoflavones that he has repeatedly suggested that soy isoflavones represent a clear and advantageous alternative to HRT.

Taking Dr. Burke's Research Seriously

Not all women will be helped with either HRT or isoflavone supplements. However, given the evidence to date, I believe that soy isoflavones represent a significant breakthrough for women who are experiencing menopausal symptoms. Isoflavones from soy can be taken by women for whom HRT is contraindicated in many cases, and such women are advised to discuss the soy isoflavone option with their family physician or gynecologist. Despite the flurry of attention given to the "miracle" of hormone therapy, a large percentage of postmenopausal women are not using it. My advice is, try soy isoflavones first. Avoid HRT when soy isoflavones are available, and effective, for you.

Unfortunately, millions of women do not know they have an alternative; to date, little is being done to educate them. What is becoming clear is that women should not be faced with only two choices, to take HRT or to do nothing at all. Given, as well, what we know about soy and its potential to help prevent cardiovascular disease and osteoporosis, it appears that a woman who decides against HRT does not have to resign herself to brittle bones or clogged arteries. Isoflavones may be the first comprehensive and safe treatment for the symptoms of menopause and for the diseases which endanger postmenopausal women. I recommend that women consult the information in this book about soy and cardiovascular disease and osteoporosis.

Are Isoflavones Safe?

Any dietary supplement (nutriceutical) is subject to misuse, just as any prescription drug is potentially dangerous. For this reason, I recommend taking isoflavone supplements for menopause at recommended dosages with the supervision of a health-care professional. This is particularly important if HRT is used concomitantly. Although isoflavone toxicity has occasionally been produced in animal studies, it has never been reported in human studies. Still, caution is the best policy. At this time, taking 50 to 100 mg of isoflavones a day is a very safe dosage for most people, considering that individuals in Asia can easily consume in excess of 100 mg or more a day from dietary sources. This dosage falls within the range used for human research purposes, and no adverse effects have ever been reported from the many studies that have been done on isoflavones. Even though soy foods are healthful for children and pregnant women, I do not recommend that pregnant women or children take isoflavones at high doses.

Isoflavone supplements are available in health food stores; they have been produced in capsule format (such as Phyto-Est) or in powdered drink mixes (such as FemSoy). These products are formulated to deliver about 50 to 60 mgs of isoflavones per day.

A discussion of consuming isoflavones in the form of a dietary supplement is in no way intended to discourage you from adding soy foods to your daily diet. Numerous books on the market (listed in the Recommended Reading List) provide literally hundreds of recipes that use soy products. From tofu-based breakfast drinks to soybean pumpkin pie to simply pouring soy milk over your breakfast cereal, the possibilities for adding soy products to your diet are endless. The health benefits of a diet that features soy foods on a regular basis are too abundant to ignore, so I encourage you to begin experimenting with the many nutritious and delicious soy products currently on the market. Nonetheless, to ensure a stable and predictable dosage of soy isoflavones, dietary supplements are recommended.

Can Soy Isoflavones Be Taken with HRT?

To date, there are no controlled studies that have examined the concomitant use of soy isoflavones and HRT. However, many women have increased their consumption of soy products—particularly soy milk, tofu, and soy isoflavone supplements—while taking HRT, and there is no record of any untoward effects. In fact, there are anecdotal reports from clinicians who have observed that adding soy to the diet of menopausal and post-menopausal women taking HRT prevents the need for high doses of the synthetic hormones. Some "bolder" physicians, those with an open mind about nutritional therapies, have substituted soy for HRT.

Clearly, more research is needed in this area. For example, we know that calcium is synergistic with HRT in promoting the health of the bones. There is some evidence that isoflavones demonstrate the same effect. Studies conducted by Dr. J. W. Erdman and his colleagues at the University of Illinois have shown unequivocally that supplementing the diet with soy protein containing isoflavones can treat osteoporosis by increasing bone density in women with post-menopausal bone loss. For mature women, I see an advantage in combining soy isoflavones with their regular calcium supplements.

IS SOY ALL YOU NEED?

Menopause is a complex issue and no single nutrient is a panacea, guaranteed to alleviate every symptom. Hormonal replacement therapy is not a cure-all either. However, maintaining a healthful diet that emphasizes plant protein, and engaging in an exercise program are both important components of preventing or easing menopausal symptoms. While exercise and its benefits for women in the perimenopausal years has not yet been extensively studied, some evidence of its benefits exist. In one study, 6 percent of women who were physically active reported experiencing hot flashes as compared with 25 percent of women who did not engage in an exercise program. Anecdotal reports certainly support the contention that exercise contributes to both physical and mental well-being. Since there is evidence that both plant-based diets (particularly soy diets) and exercise aid in the prevention of heart disease and osteoporosis, their benefits obviously extend beyond preventing specific menopausal symptoms.

Herbal therapies are also available, but I do not recommend that you experiment with them on your own because many herbal preparations have potentially serious side effects. For example, black cohosh, a plant that is a member of the buttercup family, has been shown to reduce menopausal symptoms; however, its estrogenic effect can actually aggravate existing problems with heavy menstrual flow. Its potential side effects also include dizziness, headaches, and nausea. In Germany, where black cohosh is a popular therapy for menopausal symptoms, a governmental regulatory group limits the use of black cohosh products to six months because its long-term safety has not been determined. This is not to say that herbal therapies are not useful. They are coming into wide use among health-conscious individuals, but I recommend that you seek guidance from qualified practitioners rather than experiment with herbal products on your own. In my 1998 book, *Miracle Herbs*, I discuss important issues in herbal therapy, including the standardization of herbal extracts.

Traditional Chinese medicine offers herbal formulations and acupuncture to relieve menopausal symptoms and to help regulate hormonal function. It is not surprising that practitioners of Chinese medicine may also recommend adding soy foods to the diet as part of a treatment plan. Here, too, I recommend seeking help from a qualified, licensed practitioner.

Most of the medical and self-help books about menopause currently on the market recommend lifestyle changes, such as adding effective stress management strategies (*i.e.*, exercise programs, adequate rest, and meditation or relaxation exercises). This advice is wise for men and women of any age, and I certainly agree with these authors. Most of these books also discuss improving the diet. Considering the risk factors involved with HRT, adding soy foods to your diet and taking isoflavone supplements at appropriate levels (about 50 to 80 mg per day) may be one of the best ways to use nature's pharmacy to alleviate the symptoms of menopause. I suggest that you share the thoughts presented in this book with your physician.

SOY ISOFLAVONES AND THE "NEW" ESTROGENS

A new class of drugs that offers a different type of HRT is already receiving attention in the popular press. Called SERMs—selective estrogen receptor modulators—this class of drugs mimic estrogen. An example is a drug called raloxifene, produced by Eli

Lilly and Company. It is ironic that the action of this new drug is remarkably similar to soy isoflavones.

To reiterate the earlier comparisons of soy isoflavones and raloxifene is useful at this juncture. Raloxifene is said to prevent bone loss from the hip and spine and increase bone density, a commendable feature. However, the purported increase in bone density of 2 to 3 percent with raloxifene may be less than that achievable with soy isoflavones. Raloxifene also reduced "bad" cholesterol—LDL—but so do isoflavones, which also increase good cholesterol—HDL. Soy isoflavones have been shown to relieve some menopausal symptoms, most notably hot flashes. Raloxifene does not offer this benefit. Raloxifene offers no hope of preventing Alzheimer's disease, but estrogen replacement therapy (ERT), and perhaps soy isoflavones, may protect against Alzheimer's.

All in all, SERMs do not seem to offer anything that improves upon soy isoflavones. But SERMs are synthetic drugs and, there-fore, can be protected by patents and proprietary interests. Con-sumers, however, have a choice. They can use isoflavones, which have been safely consumed for centuries, or they can choose a synthetic formulation that offers similar benefits. The sensible choice here is the remedy of natural origin.

WHAT ABOUT PREMENSTRUAL SYNDROME?

In discussing soy and menopause, I do not want to ignore the syndrome known as premenstrual syndrome (PMS). The trouble-some symptoms many women experience with this syndrome are related to hormone imbalance. Some women are miserable for two or three days prior to menstrual flow; a minority of women report symptoms for seven to fourteen days, with the intensity of the symptoms increasing from about the time of ovulation to the beginning of the menstrual flow.

To date, there is no "concrete" evidence that a soy-based diet will prevent the symptoms of PMS. However, anecdotal observations imply a potential benefit. It is worth postulating that the estrogenic effects of soy isoflavones could be beneficial during certain phases of the menstrual cycle when the effects of estrogen fluctuate.

There is scientific evidence that consuming soy milk and soy protein can increase the length of the menstrual cycle in adult females. Supplementing the diet with soy had a variable effect on levels of the estrogenic hormone estradiol as well as on other hormones that regulate menstruation, including luteinizing hormone (LH), progesterone, follicle stimulating hormone (FSH), and dehydroepiandrosterone (DHEA).

It would seem that increasing intake of soy isoflavones to levels similar to those consumed in soy-based diets—about 50 to 80 mg per day—is a safe option. This can be accomplished by adding soy foods to the diet and using isoflavone nutritional supplements. I do not recommend taking higher doses because the safety (for humans) of isoflavones in doses over 120 mg a day is unknown, especially in the long term.

In general, the recommendations for coping with menopause and PMS are quite similar. A diet that emphasizes plant proteins and other complex carbohydrates combined with a regular exercise program usually go a long way to prevent—and alleviate—many of the difficulties associated with menstruation.

ANDROPAUSE— THE MALE AT MID-LIFE

The manifestations of male andropause are not as obvious and overt as they are in the female menopause. In the fields of medicine, psychology, and even social psychology, there are those who do not acknowledge the phenomenon of andropause. Nonetheless, the male biological clock is influenced by hormonal changes, and it is not a myth that a male who is approximately fifty years of age (or somewhere between thirty-five and sixty-five) can go through physical and psychosocial changes that have much in common to those experienced by females during the climacteric. It is time that we stopped confusing the andropause with "mid-life" crisis. The so-called mid-life crisis may occur in both sexes for many reasons but, except for coinciding chronologically, be unrelated to andropause or menopause.

Both the menopause and andropause represent large-scale movements of the biological clock. Just as the menopause is precipitated by the relative lack of estrogen and progesterone, the dominant female hormones, the andropause is associated with the declining availability of the male sex hormone testosterone. There is, however, no clear definable event to mark the occurrence of andro-pause. The waning of the influences of testosterone during andropause occurs much more slowly than the relatively abrupt cessation of estrogen and progesterone that occurs with menopause.

It is commonly stated that men may age better than women. One of the reasons for this could be the fact that when testosterone starts to exert less influence, the mature male may become relatively feminized. By feminization, I do not mean obvious or extensive physical changes—just that, to some degree, the body tissues in the mature male may become less responsive to the effects of testosterone.

Several clearly recognizable changes can be attributed to testosterone deficiency in the male. These include lack of exercise tolerance, change in body shape, lessening of sexual drive, changes in psychological well-being, skin changes, and urogenital changes. Reduction in secondary sex characteristics, such as loss of facial or body hair, and poor sexual performance may also occur. These are the areas in which many men may suffer in silence.

Unfortunately, there are no clearly defined or accepted hormonal interventions for men. I believe that there may be hundreds of thousands of men who have visited health care providers with symptoms of the andropause, but they have been passed off as merely showing signs of "normal" aging. It is possible for the male with andropause to appear physically fit on clinical examination; subtle clinical signs of the andropause, such as loss of body hair or testicular softening, may not be obvious to the examining physician. Even if the practitioner considers the andropause a definable condition, there are no "clear-cut" laboratory procedures for defining the biochemical changes that can result in the diagnosis of the andropause. The measurement of blood levels of testosterone can assist in detecting the more gross cases of androgen insufficiency, but the lack of correlation between testosterone levels and all andropausal symptoms makes the diagnosis of andropause very difficult.

The real risk is that the andropausal male, who could respond to an intervention such as testosterone replacement therapy, instead finds himself on the receiving end of inappropriate medical advice or treatment. Antidepressant drugs, tranquilizers, or sedatives are often prescribed, but these may actually worsen the situation for an andropausal male. These types of drugs are commonly used in psychiatric practice, but they may amplify the changes experienced in andropause. A male with declining libido runs the risk of being turned into an impotent male as a consequence of inappropriate drug therapy.

SOY AND A HEALTHY PROSTATE GLAND

Prostatic disease will affect almost every man who lives long enough. There are approximately 125,000 new cases of prostate cancer per year in the United States, and the incidence increases in men with each decade after age fifty. Benign prostate disease is also a concern. The causes of benign enlargement of the prostate (BPH) remain uncertain but, like prostate cancer, it appears to involve hormonal imbalances that occur with aging. (Refer to Chapter 7, which includes a discussion of the prostate and the prevention of both benign and malignant prostatic diseases.) I urge you to discuss these important issues with your health-care provider.

I believe that the growing population of men and women who are now moving into their mid-life years will increasingly rely on improved diet and remedies of natural origin for maintenance of good health. Soy, in both dietary and supplemental form, offers a nutrient with well-tested health-giving properties that particularly promotes health at this stage of life.

CHAPTER 10

Thinning Bones and Creaky Joints May Not Be Inevitable

Bones are living tissue, with their continuing health dependent on the nutrients you ingest and absorb. The body has an intricate mechanism to both form new bone tissue and dispose of damaged tissue. *Osteoblasts* are the cells involved in forming new bone tissue; *osteoclasts* are cells that model, or break down, damaged or old bone tissue in a process known as *resorption*. Bone mass, the amount of mineral in our bones, reaches its peak between the ages of thirty and thirty-five. After that it begins to decline naturally. However, this decline too often turns into the progressive disease of osteoporosis. Untold suffering and disability results from osteoporosis, the gradual thinning of bone tissue that results in porous, brittle bones. The disease occurs in both men and women, although women are considered much more at risk than men.

People suffering from advancing osteoporosis are vulnerable to some specific types of fractures. The first, the spontaneous vertebral crush fracture, occurs when one of the spinal vertebrae weakens to the point that it may collapse under minimal stress, even one's own body weight. Repeated crush fractures lead to loss of height but, even more serious, the ability of the spine to support upright stature is compromised. The hunched over posture of an elderly person who may need a cane or a walker for balance is a characteristic sign that a vertebral crush fracture has occurred.

Caucasian women who are small-boned and fair-skinned tend to be in a high-risk group. An individual's genetic profile, overall health, and lifestyle also influence risk. Cigarette smoking, excessive coffee or cola intake, and excessive alcohol consumption are also considered risk factors for later development of osteoporosis. For purposes of our discussion, however, virtually everyone is at risk and should be concerned about skeletal health and the increased incidence—and risk—of bone fractures among the elderly. With a bit of luck, we are all going to live longer, and mobility as we get older is worth fighting for.

ADVANCING AGE MAY BE JUST PART OF THE STORY

Age-adjusted studies performed in the last two or three decades have demonstrated that factors other than normal aging are involved in the rising rate of osteoporosis. For one thing, not all of the world's populations appear to have the same vulnerability to the disease. People in the West tend to have higher incidence of osteoporosis, even though their intake of calcium is much higher than that of most other population groups.

This demographic information imposes a need to look outside aging for causes of this disease, particularly since the information also indicates a decrease in overall health of bone tissue throughout our population. Osteoporosis does have links with other medical conditions, particularly those involving the endocrine system. Diabetes as well as conditions affecting the thyroid or adrenal glands may be factors in thinning of the bones. Persons taking corticosteroid drugs and some common prescription medications, including lithium and other psychotropic drugs, also have increased risk of bone loss.

CALCIUM ALONE IS NOT THE ANSWER

No doubt you learned at an early age that calcium is responsible for building strong bones and teeth. This is certainly true, but it is only part of the picture. Your bones require varying amounts of numerous minerals, as well as protein, to develop and maintain their structural integrity. When they are healthy, your bones have the ability to repair minor fractures, often caused by stress and bone fatigue, and you may not be aware that you have had such an injury. In addition, the remodeling process itself is designed to increase a bone's ability to meet the stress and demands made on it.

An example of how this works is the way the long bones in the legs of professional dancers become thicker and stronger from the stress placed on them. This is the body's way of adapting, and is, at least in part, the thinking behind advising women to engage in weight-bearing exercise both before and after menopause. (Preventing osteoporosis is, of course, only one of the many benefits of exercise for both men and women of any age.)

Calcium Intake

Current emphasis in treatment is on increasing calcium intake. Some research studies also have shown that a multi-nutrient approach that features calcium is beneficial both for treatment and for prevention of the disease; one study in particular demonstrated that calcium therapy reduced vertebral crush fractures among postmenopausal women by about 50 percent.

Millions of Western women are augmenting their diets with calcium supplements, sometimes taking in excess of 1,500 milligrams per day. However, there is a threshold for the amount of calcium the body can absorb and efficiently use. Excessive calcium intake may, under certain circumstances, create health problems. The Recommended Daily Allowance is a sensible guide to optimal calcium requirements. (See Table 8, based on the National Institutes of Health Consensus Statement.)

TABLE 8
OPTIMAL CALCIUM REQUIREMENTS
DURING AN INDIVIDUAL'S LIFETIME*

Stage of Life	Optimal daily intake (in mg of calcium)
Women	
25-50 years	1000
Pregnant and nursing	1200-15009
Over 50 years (postmenopausal)	
On estrogens	1000
Not on estrogens	1500
Over 65 years	1500
Men	
25-65 years	1000
Over 65 years	1500
Adolescents/young adults	
11-24 years	1200-1500
Children	
Up to 10 years 800-1200	
Infants	
Up to 1 year	400-600

*Data modified from NIH Consensus Statement, Vol. 12, No. 4, June 6-8, 1994.

Since menopause is not a single event, but a process that occurs over a period of years, some thinning of the bones takes place prior to cessation of menstruation. Thus, it is critical that women maintain an optimal calcium intake before, during, and after menopause. Studies further suggest that it is important to concentrate on preventing the rapid bone loss that occurs during the five to ten years following the last menstrual period. The more difficult decision for many women, then, is whether they should use estrogen replacement therapy as a means to prevent bone loss during this critical postmenopausal period. Once menopause is over, many women are advised to keep taking replacement hormones in order to prevent heart disease, as well as osteoporosis.

I worry about the risks of long-term HRT for mature women. Taking a calcium supplement is one thing, but life-long estrogen replacement is another issue. To be sure, as a dual treatment, calcium supplements and estrogen replacement have demonstrably decreased bone loss among postmenopausal women. However, we always need to consider the risks of hormone replacement and weigh them against the benefits. As we saw when the subject of estrogen replacement therapy came up before, when there are questions about its long-term risks, it makes sense to consider an alternative. I suggest that the phytoestrogens found in soybeans may be a safe and adequate treatment for many women who do not choose to use synthetic estrogens. Soy can help the body retain calcium and maintain the integrity of the bones.

TABLE 9
RELATIONSHIP BETWEEN CALCIUM INTAKE AND
HIP FRACTURE RATE IN VARIOUS COUNTRIES*

Country	Calcium intake (approximate mg/day)	Hip fracture rate (per 100,000 people)
South Africa (blacks)	196	6.8
Hong Kong	356	45.6
Singapore	389	21.6
New Guinea	448	3.1
Yugoslavia	588	27.6
Spain	766	42.4
Israel	794	93.2
Denmark	960	165.3
United States	973	144.9
United Kingdom	977	118.2
Holland	1,006	87.7
Norway	1,087	190.4
Sweden	1,104	187.8
Ireland	1,110	76.0
New Zealand	1,217	119.0
Finland	1,332	111.2

*Note the high rate of hip fractures in countries where calcium intake is higher (Messina and Messina, 1994).

HOW DOES SOY HELP PREVENT OSTEOPOROSIS?

As we pointed out earlier, people in Western countries consume much more calcium than the rest of the world. Yet they have a higher risk of osteoporosis. For example, hip fractures among the elderly are far more common in the United Kingdom, the United States, and Scandinavian countries than they are among the Black population of South Africa or the Chinese population in Hong Kong (note table). The mystery of why this happens may be fairly easily solved when we consider that Western countries also con-

TABLE 10
RELATIONSHIP BETWEEN ANIMAL PROTEIN INTAKE AND HIP FRACTURE RATE IN VARIOUS COUNTRIES*

Country	Animal protein intake (approximate g/day)	Hip fracture rate (per 100,000 people)
South Africa (blacks)	10.4	6.8
New Guinea	16.4	3.1
Singapore	24.7	21.6
Yugoslavia	27.3	27.6
Hong Kong	34.6	45.6
Israel	42.5	93.2
Spain	47.6	42.4
Holland	54.3	87.7
United Kingdom	56.6	118.2
Denmark	58.0	165.3
Sweden	59.4	187.8
Finland	60.5	111.2
Ireland	61.4	76.0
Norway	66.6	190.4
United States	72.0	144.9
New Zealand	77.8	119.0

*From Messina and Messina, 1994.

sume more animal protein. There is an adage, "It's not what you make, it's what you keep." It appears that a variation on this adage applies to calcium and animal protein. The simple fact is that diets high in animal protein promote loss of calcium through the urine (hypercalciuria).

On the other hand, soy protein has a calcium sparing effect, meaning that soy helps the body retain a greater amount of ingested calcium. This information does not negate the importance of including adequate calcium in the diet, but it demonstrates that calcium retention is an issue that needs more attention than it has been given thus far.

Moreover, when calcium intake is inadequate in the first place, then urinary losses take an even larger toll on skeletal health. Discovering the link between excessive protein consumption and loss of calcium through the urine leads us to conclude that we have found one of the most important factors in the high incidence of osteoporosis in the Western world.

Important studies, published in the late 1980s, examined the relationship between animal protein-rich diets and calcium metabolism, especially as it relates to the formation of kidney stones. Three groups were studied: one group consumed protein derived from meat and cheese; another group consumed protein from cheese, eggs, soy milk, and texturized vegetable protein; and a third group consumed protein solely from soy products. The first group lost 50 percent more calcium in their urine than the third group, the one that consumed only soy protein. Within the second group, calcium loss was greater, but not as great as in the group that consumed meat and cheese.

This study is significant because it reinforces the benefits of adding soy protein to the diet for the purpose of preventing calcium loss. In a very real sense, it helps you to understand that *retaining* the calcium you ingest is more important than the absolute number of milligrams you include in your diet or through supplements. These findings have been confirmed through animal studies, which also demonstrated that soy protein-rich diets delayed age-related bone loss and reduced the total amount of bone loss. At this point, consuming soy protein can legitimately be viewed as a strong potential tool in the prevention of osteoporosis.

Some soy milk products are fortified with calcium and vitamin D, and soy milk also contains isoflavones. Dr. Chai-Won Chung is a pediatrician who has devoted much of his life to developing soy beverages, including soy infant formulas. A product called Vegemil A, is an adult soy beverage developed by Dr. Chung's Soyfood Company, Ltd., in Korea. Fortified with calcium and vitamin D, it is a particularly attractive dietary option for bone health because soy isoflavones and calcium occur together.

Calcilum and Soy Work Together

The reasons why soy protein has a protective effect against calcium loss are not entirely clear. However, the amino acid content of soy is probably involved. Soy protein tends to be low in sulfur-containing amino acids, which are believed to promote hypercalciuria. There is no question that calcium is essential to prevent osteoporosis, along with regular exercise and a lifestyle free of smoking and alcohol consumption. The ideal scenario is to consume soy protein along with calcium, which is possible with supplementation or by consuming a small or moderate amount of dairy products if desired. However, for consumers—particularly women—who choose to avoid dairy products for other reasons, calcium supplements and soy protein offer a viable and attractive alternative.

Soy protein fortified with calcium, in the form of a supplemental powder, may be the most convenient way to gain the benefits of both calcium and soy. Remember, too, that soybeans do contain some calcium, and the National Institutes of Health have mentioned calcium-containing soy products as a good source of dietary calcium. In my opinion, the value of soy isoflavones and calcium make soy milk, fortified with calcium and vitamin D, a more attractive drink than dairy milk.

A WORD ABOUT CALCIUM SUPPLEMENTS

Calcium supplements come in many formulas. A common one is inorganic calcium salts, but these supplements may have absorption that is unpredictable and may interfere with iron absorption as well. Calcium carbonate is more commonly recommended because of its higher percentage of available calcium per tablet. It is produced in massive quantities for the Western market.

Calcium supplements will continue to play an important role in preventing and treating osteoporosis, and available research supports supplementation. However, with our knowledge of the benefits of soy and the results of Dr. Erdman's research studies before us, it is obvious that calcium supplements need to be complemented with soy protein and isoflavones. The addition of nutrient-rich soy products provides an important tool in promoting the healthiest bones possible.

SOY AND ARTHRITIS

Osteoporosis and osteoarthritis are so closely linked that it is hard to find evidence of one without the other. Osteoarthritis, the most common type of arthritis, at its onset is typically not associated with marked inflammation. It is popularly referred to as "wear and tear" arthritis. Rheumatoid arthritis is usually more severe and crippling, commonly resulting in deformity.

All forms of advanced arthritis have unwanted blood vessel growth as part of their progression. This unwanted blood vessel growth occurs in and around the joint, and a "vascular pannus" (inflammatory mass) can occur. The soy isoflavones daidzein and genistein are antiangiogenic, meaning that they can interfere with unwanted blood vessel growth around arthritic joints. Researchers have reported a clear association between inhibition of new blood vessel growth and improvement in the symptoms of osteoarthritis.

Recently the importance of omega-3 fatty acids in the treatment of rheumatoid arthritis has been highlighted in the medical literature. Soy foods contain precursors to omega-3 fatty acids, and this may account for some of the anecdotal reports of the benefits of soy-based diets for some people with rheumatoid arthritis. It appears that soy has many properties that can promote both bone and joint health.

Soy and Cancer

Cancer is neither one disease nor one process. Rather, it takes many forms and its development involves many processes. These processes often begin with an initiating event. For example, a carcinogenic substance is introduced into the body—a substance that has the potential to damage the body's cells—and, at some point, triggers the development of a form of cancer. You might be thinking that if we developed cancer every time a carcinogen entered our bodies, our species would have become extinct long ago. You are right. The body's defense system is a network of complex interactions that is designed to mount a very powerful defense against invaders such as microorganisms that cause disease and chemicals that cause cancer. We are only beginning to understand how it works, but we do know that the immune system is important in fighting cancer. In fact, the research about protecting the body and preventing various types of cancer from developing in the first place is truly the most exciting area of information currently coming in on the struggle to conquer this disease.

A CHAIN OF EVENTS

A carcinogen can damage a cell and result in cancer only when the cell is awakened by circumstances that encourages it to divide. We can think of this as a situation in which some damaged cells are asleep; they do no harm because they do not bother other cells. When the cells become active, however, they begin to damage the cells around them.

In the most simple terms, cancer prevention is a process of minimizing damage to the cells, or keeping damaged, dormant cells inactive, or even changing them back to normal. It is safe to say that we are all subject to the initiating stage of cancer as we are all exposed to carcinogenic agents, from exhaust fumes to ultraviolet rays to toxic metals. We can attempt to minimize our exposure, but we can't live in protective bubbles. Our best chance is to interfere with the "awakening" or "promoting" stage of cancer by adopting the right lifestyle.

Cancer	*Premalignant Conditions*	*Screening Process*
Esophagus	Barrett's epithelium	Endoscopy with biopsy
Colon	Adenomatous polyp	Fecal occult-blood test, endoscopy
Breast	Intraductal, preinvasive, cancer	Self examination screening mammogram
Cervix	Dysplasia of varying grade	Cervical Smear
Bladder cancer	Polyps in bladder	Urine testing, Cystoscopy
Uterus cancer	Preinvasive cancer	Curettage
Lung	Dysplasia of the bronchial epithelium	Chest x-ray bronchoscopy

CHANGING LOCATION, CHANGING DIET

Studies about cancer rates across large populations have demonstrated that breast cancer rates in Asia are significantly lower than in the West. During this century, significant numbers of people have moved from Asia to the United States and other Western countries. However, within two generations or so, the women in these immigrant groups have the same breast cancer rates as American women of European-American descent. Given these data, genetic predisposition is unlikely to tell the whole story. Rather, the data suggest that environmental issues are at work. One obvious factor to look at is diet and nutrition. Soybeans play an important dietary role in Japan and China, but once on U.S. soil, the Asian immigrant diet usually begins to change; within a generation or two, Japanese and Chinese Americans are eating a typical American diet with little or no soybeans. Both breast and prostate cancer rates reflect the dietary changes.

Studying men and prostate cancer provided the same clues as with breast cancer, supporting the hypothesis that soy has an important part to play in protecting the body from this disease. A group of men of Japanese ancestry living in Hawaii were studied over a twenty-year period, and the incidence of prostate cancer was substantially less among those who consumed tofu regularly. To break it down in more detail, the men who consumed tofu once a week or less were three times more likely to develop prostate cancer when compared with those who ate tofu daily. In this case, tofu, a specific soy product, was found to be the most protective food.

Other studies have investigated colon and stomach cancers, and the research adds credibility to the link between soy and cancer prevention. For example, a study performed in China showed that those who consumed soy milk had a significantly lower chance of developing stomach cancer than those who didn't include this food in their diets. Another Chinese study confirmed that those who included soy (not only soy milk) in their diets reduced their risk of stomach cancer by 40 percent. A study of Japanese-Hawaiians found that those who included tofu in their diets reduced their risk of colon cancer by one third.

Japanese studies suggest that soy reduced the risk of rectal cancer by 80 percent and colon cancer by 40 percent. It was concluded that even relatively low levels of soy consumption provided measurable cancer protection. The American Cancer Society now considers colo-rectal cancer preventable, and researchers in the United States have begun taking population studies seriously that link dietary habits to cancer formation. This information can no longer be dismissed or simply ignored.

FROM POPULATION STUDIES TO THE LAB

Science requires more than epidemiological data to make definitive statements. We could look at these population studies and make broad recommendations that soy should be a part of every diet, but for such recommendations to have real credibility they have to be based on the kind of proof that science demands. When we test animals, however, we are able to use the lab to completely control the conditions of the test, something we cannot effectively do with humans. Mark and Virginia Messina have summarized a series of studies performed on animals that demonstrated the anticancer effects of soy-based diets. They reported these studies in their book, *The Simple Soybean and Your Health*.

Among the most important studies are those conducted at the University of Alabama by Stephen Barnes and his colleagues. Reported a few years ago, these studies showed that adding modest amounts of soy products to laboratory rat feed provided protection against cancer formation. The evidence was so clear that it caused a major stir in the scientific community and also increased the public's curiosity about soy. Many other animal studies show a cancer-protective role for soy and soy isoflavones.

When we combine data collected in epidemiological and animal studies, we can only conclude that there is a credible body of evidence that strongly suggests that the simple soybean plant shows great anticancer properties. Still, many questions remain. What is it about soy that protects against cancer? Are there pecific chemicals at work, and should we simply view all soy products and derivatives as the same?

A FAMILY OF SUBSTANCES TO EXPLORE

Among the most widely discussed substances found in soybeans are isoflavones. If you remember, isoflavones are included among the many classes of flavonoids and are phytoestrogens—plant estrogens. Plant estrogens were once believed to be potentially harmful to humans because their action in the body was misunderstood. Essentially, we now know that while isoflavones are chemically similar to estrogens produced in the body, their effects are weaker.

What this means for soy and cancer prevention can be illustrated by the case of breast tumors that are estrogen-sensitive. When natural estrogen binds with estrogen receptor sites in cells in the breast it stimulates cell division. If a latent tumor is present, estrogen may trigger its growth. Estrogen is a cancer promoter in these circumstances, and for this reason, some chemotherapeutic agents are designed to curtail the effects of natural estrogens circulating through the body. However, when isoflavones bind with estrogen receptor sites they prevent the more potent form of estrogen from affecting the cell. Thus isoflavones accomplish the same task as the chemotherapeutic agents are designed to do, but isoflavones do it without the side effects that directly attacking the body's natural estrogen with chemotherapeutic agents causes.

The Tamoxifen Story

Tamoxifen is a drug used to treat breast cancer that functions somewhat like isoflavones do. It binds with estrogen receptors

TABLE 11
BREAST CANCER MORTALITY IN SOY FOOD-CONSUMING
COUNTRIES COMPARED WITH THE UNITED STATES

Country	Soy Intake/g/day	Breast cancer rate	Prostate cancer rate
Japan	29.5	6.0	3.5
Korea	19.9	2.6	0.5
Hong Kong	10.3	8.4	2.9
China	9.3	4.7	Unknown
United States	Negligible	22.4	15.7

Rates are age adjusted; deaths are per 100,000 people.

and keeps the "fertilizer-like" estrogen from moving in and promoting cell growth. Tamoxifen had been used for twenty years in the treatment of breast cancer when results of a new study of its effectiveness for prevention of breast cancer were released in the spring of 1998, to a lot of publicity. Dr. Richard Klausner, director of the National Cancer Institute, reported that a randomized, controlled trial of tamoxifen in almost 14,000 women at risk for cancer found that the rate of breast cancer occurrence was cut by about one half in the women who took tamoxifen, compared with the women in the study who took a placebo.

This was good news, but it was clouded by also having to announce that tamoxifen has some very sinister side effects. The women taking tamoxifen experienced a third more blood clots and more than twice as many cases of cancer of the uterus as the placebo group did, and they were not the only side effects mentioned—only the most important. When physicians begin to offer healthy people a drug with such serious potential side effects, on the chance it will prevent another disease, it could be time to remind them of Hippocrates's famous admonition to physicians to "above all, do no harm."

The need to accept such risk might be a little easier to understand if there were no alternatives, but an examination of soy and its phytoestrogens, genistein and daidzein, quickly reveals that there are. Like tamoxifen, these soy fractions lock on to estrogen receptors in the breast, functioning as an antiestrogen in that part of the body while they also function as an estrogen in the blood to prevent bone loss and lower cholesterol. On the other hand, soy phytoestrogens do not cause cancer of the uterus and, instead of fostering the formation of blood clots, they are known to inhibit platelet aggregation in the blood—they inhibit blood clots.

It really is too bad that these facts about the effectiveness of soy cannot be announced with the same fanfare that tamoxifen received. Perhaps when the National Cancer Institute finally becomes willing to advance the kind of resources for a study of soy phytoestrogens that they provided for a prevention study of a twenty-year-old drug that was already well known to prevent breast cancer from recurring in women, perhaps then such fanfare will come to soy.

MEN ARE AFFECTED BY HORMONALLY STIMULATED CANCERS, TOO

Cancers can grow at a rapid rate and overwhelm the body quickly; conversely, they sometimes grow for many years before effects on the body are manifest. Researchers have noted, for instance, that Japanese men may develop prostate cancer, but because it grows so slowly, it often does not become a killer disease. Instead the men who have it die of other causes before their prostate cancer develops symptoms or spreads to surrounding lymph nodes and bones. The discovery by Japanese researchers in the 1980s that the soy isoflavone genistein can block the signal that triggers the growth of cancer cells seems to explain this phenomenon.

As I have said, cancer is a disease that involves a chain of events. One such event is the activation of compounds such as epidermal growth factor (EGF), which is involved in cell growth and division. Certain enzymes, including tyrosine kinases, can stimulate and activate EGF; it appears that genistein inhibits or blocks tyrosine kinases. Therefore, genistein can interrupt the signal that causes cancer cells to grow.

Instead of "attacking" cancer cells and obliterating them, genistein acts here in a more subtle but no less effective way. People tend to think of cancer prevention and treatment as a war in which "good" substances fight the "bad" cancer cells and wipe them out. However, sometimes the real story—the real miracle—if you will, is less like a war and more like a negotiation. This occurs when the body is able to protect itself against the activation of a cancer or is able to inhibit the cancer's growth to the extent that the body is not significantly harmed. This "battle," which is really a delicate balancing act, has been going on since the beginning of life on our planet.

CANCER AND MODULATING ANGIOGENESIS

The process of vascularization, or forming new blood vessels, is essential for the healing of wounds and repair of tissue. However, known as angiogenesis, it also plays a major role in the propagation of several disease states, including cancer. Dr. Judah Folkman of the Massachusetts Institute of Technology is credited with the discovery of the importance of angiogenesis in tumor development. The onset of angiogenic activity appears to occur as a definable event in tumor formation, and most solid tumors depend at some point on the development of tumor circulation, which requires blood vessels (vascularization). It is logical, therefore, to attempt to inhibit the growth of these new blood vessels, thereby stopping or limiting the growth of the tumor.

The importance of angiogenesis in the promotion of cancer growth has fueled a considerable amount of research into control of its mechanism. Tumor angiogenesis factors (TAF) have been identified and a flurry of research has identified agents and cofactors that inhibit—or modulate—angiogenesis. Some interesting information has already emerged about the potential antiangiogenic actions of soy isoflavones. In animal studies the isoflavone genistein blocked angiogenesis and was found to have direct tumoricidal properties against several tumor types. It also regulated key enzyme expression, a process involved in tumor growth. Genistein is obviously a very strong candidate for further investigation as an antiangiogenic agent in humans.

THE ALL-IMPORTANT ANTIOXIDANTS

Just over a decade ago, most lay people had never heard of antioxidants; however, in recent years research has confirmed their role in cancer prevention. Antioxidant substances protect the body against the harmful effects of free radicals—renegade oxygen molecules that damage membranes in cells and trigger mutations in DNA, the material found in the chromosomes that holds genetic information in the cells. Mutations in DNA cause various aberrations, including cancer.

Vitamins C and E are well-known antioxidants. Phytic acid, though less well-known, is also a very powerful antioxidant. Found only in plant foods such as grains, nuts, and legumes, it protects seeds against free radicals and helps preserve them and extend their life. Soybeans are rich in phytic acid. (Unsprouted soy seeds have been known to survive for hundreds of years.)

Phytic acid is a chelating agent, which simply means that its molecules are capable of binding to metals. Binding metals is an essential action of antioxidants. Phytic acid is one substance that binds easily with iron. When iron is exposed to oxygen, free radicals can be created, which in turn threaten the DNA of cells. Phytic acid binds with iron and keeps it away from oxygen, thus preventing damage. Certain soy-based foods, such as tempeh and miso, have been studied as potential free-radical scavengers, meaning that they are important in maintaining efficient operation of body defenses against cancer.

Scientists know that potential carcinogens can be produced through food processing and cooking. For example, when beef is fried at high temperatures, a number of mutagenic—that is, potentially carcinogenic substances—are produced. But adding ten percent soy protein to fried ground beef prevented production of these mutagenic agents. We have known for a long time that potential carcinogens in foods are virtually impossible to avoid, but it is exciting indeed to think that we have begun to establish unequivocally that soy foods provide a protection against these cancer-causing agents in other foods.

SOY'S ROLE IN PREVENTING COLON CANCER

Digestion is extremely complex, and a full discussion of the way food is broken down and nutrients absorbed is outside the scope of this book. However, one particular component of digestion is influenced by soy; specifically, the bacterial flora found in the large bowel. Under normal conditions, the large bowel contains beneficial bacteria that aid in the metabolism of all the foods we eat. Certain complex sugars found in soy, such as raffinose and stachyose, provide sustenance for beneficial bacteria in the colon. Some researchers recommend supplementing the diet with these sugars to encourage the presence of the health-promoting bacteria. The aim is for beneficial bacteria to grow in the colon and displace the effects of any potentially harmful bacteria found there. We do not need large amounts of these sugars to receive their beneficial effects.

Some evidence also exists showing that soy affords protection against colon cancers by interfering with the growth of polyps (precancerous growths) in the colons of test animals. We can surmise that soybean fiber may work together with certain sugars to protect the human colon against the cancer. However, we are basing this conclusion on circumstantial evidence, and more research is still needed to learn all the details of soya's protective mechanisms here.

CHAPTER 12

Dairy Versus Soy: Is There One Answer?

As it always has, soy remains an inexpensive source of many nutritious foods in Asia and the foundation diet of many Asian societies. However, soy milk has another reason to be popular there, and that is because lactose intolerance is widespread among Asian people.

LACTOSE INTOLERANCE

Lactose is the primary sugar found in milk. It requires the presence of the enzyme lactase in the small bowel before it can be fully digested. If this enzyme is lacking, lactose will enter the colon intact; intestinal bacteria will then feed on it, producing acids and gas. This, in turn, may cause cramping, diarrhea, and flatulence.

For many Asians, therefore, soy milk is an obvious choice. However, it is probable that lactose intolerance is far more widespread outside Asia than people are aware. The estimates are that for every person who has identified their lactose intolerance, there are as many as twenty others who lack the digestive enzyme, lactase, without realizing it. I believe that lactose intolerance is one of the most commonly overlooked causes of nonspecific abdominal pain and gastrointestinal distress.

The Forgotten Cause of Stomach Aches

In their 1987 book, *The Milk Sugar Dilemma: Living with Lactose Intolereance*, Richard A. Martens and Sherlyn Martens write: "Unexplained diarrhea and/or gaseousness, especially when it occurs daily, is progressive through the waking hours, or meal related, should be considered probably caused by lactose intolerance until disproved." Potentially, this description includes many people; perhaps it fits you.

Lactose intolerance is known to be widespread among certain ethnic groups. For example, it is practically universal among Asians, adult African blacks, and Dravidian Indians. About 70 percent of African-Americans and 60-70 percent of Hispanic-Americans probably have lactose intolerance. In addition, nonspecific abdominal complaints in children are often related to lactose intolerance.

Obviously, there are many causes of gastrointestinal difficulties, and these should not be overlooked. Irritable bowel syndrome (IBS) or functional dyspepsia, for instance, are also possible diagnoses. What is disturbing, however, is that many people are given diagnostic labels such as irritable bowel syndrome without being screened for lactose intolerance. Parents might be told that their child is having "growing pains" when the simple explanation is the inability to digest lactose. Even worse, both adults and children may be advised to seek psychological help or stress management for "nervous stomach" or IBS when a simple dietary change may be in order.

Lactose is Everywhere

Lactose is present in most dairy products and even in some foods of nondairy designation. Many adults essentially self-diagnose lactose intolerance because they are able to make the connection between gastrointestinal distress and a milkshake or cheese sandwich they just ate for lunch. When this happens again and again, they conclude that they do not feel well after eating dairy and may decide to avoid these products altogether.

Nowadays, there are several ways to manage lactose intolerance without completely giving up milk products. The authors of *The Milk Sugar Dilemma* offer many solutions to manage the condition. Ingesting lactose-free dairy products and dairy products to which lactase has been added are two possible solutions. Lactase tablets are also available. These tablets essentially add the missing enzyme and are taken when dairy is consumed. Of course, dairy products made from soy milk are also available and have many benefits.

SOY MILK: THE HEALTHFUL ALTERNATIVE

Given the many health benefits of soy, it makes sense for people with lactose intolerance to avail themselves of soy products. The condition, which once may have caused them so much trouble, may actually be a blessing in disguise for those ethnic groups who are forced to adjust their diet to avoid dairy. Of course, it makes sense for those who do tolerate dairy to consume more soy foods, too.

In June of 1997, I lectured at the International Symposium on Soy Milk and Cow's Milk, hosted by the Korean Soybean Society in Seoul, South Korea. The participants in the symposium gathered to discuss the research on the nutritional benefits of soy milk and cow's milk, emphasizing the implications of both of these foods for overall health. The predominant conclusion was that soy milk is an efficient and nutritious food, which offers significant advantages over cow's milk. Soy milk appears to have the ability to counteract some of the health problems that can be attributed to excessive intake of dairy.

A long-time researcher with the U.S. Food and Drug Administration (FDA), Insu P. Lee, Ph.D., is now a technical advisor to the Korean FDA. He believes that although dairy products are legitimately implicated as a major cause of several human diseases, they are finding an increased global presence. Dr. Lee has used the term "chemopreventive" to describe a potential of soy milk to prevent many common diseases and conditions because of its many health-giving nutrients.

COW'S MILK AND INFANTS

It probably comes as no surprise to many parents that cow's milk formula is not necessarily ideal. In fact, between 10 and 30 percent of newborns and infants given formula derived from cow's milk demonstrate a variety of adverse reactions. These include: diarrhea, failure to thrive, gastroenteritis, abdominal cramps, bloating and gas, general fussiness, colic, skin rashes, eczema, spitting up, incessant crying at night, general irritability, and even vomiting and wheezing. However, some studies have shown that replacing cow's milk with soy-based formula can reduce these problems by 90 percent. Studies have also shown that eczema caused by an intolerance to cow's milk protein is reversed when a soy-based formula is substituted.

Preventing the unpleasant reactions to cow's milk formula is extremely important, but it is not the whole story. There is evidence that soy-based formulas may have nutritional advantages over cow's milk. A study comparing cow's milk formula to soy formula showed some important differences in the mineralization of bones. Mineralization means the laying down of calcium in the bones. The infants fed soy-based formula showed a higher bone mineralization after approximately four months.

Twenty years of accumulated research has given scientists a body of evidence that soy-based infant formulas can make a significant contribution to managing diarrhea, allergies, and skin rashes associated with cow's milk formula. In addition, if soy milk is introduced in early childhood it has the potential to prevent certain allergies, high blood cholesterol, childhood arthritis (and perhaps the later development of arthritis in adults), cancer, and possibly other chronic conditions. I am not recommending soy milk or cow's milk ahead of mother's milk for babies. Whenever possible, infants must be breast fed.

WHAT MAKES SOY MILK HEALTHIER THAN COW'S MILK?

The simple answer to this question lies in the overall chemical composition of soy milk. To use Dr. Lee's terminology, the chemopreventive role of soy can be attributed to a variety of agents that may be present in soy milk. For example, soy milk contains the omega-3 unsaturated essential fatty acid called linolenic acid. Linolenic acid is a precursor of the health-giving omega-3 fatty acids such as DHA (decosahexanoic acid) and EPA (eicosapeutanoic acid). Research has shown that DHA is an important "brain food" in that it promotes healthy brain function, including cognitive functions. EPA has anti-inflammatory properties and shows versatile, beneficial effects on cardiovascular functioning.

The major proteins in milk are caseins and whey proteins, which do offer significant health benefits. For example, lactoferrin, a whey protein, appears to offer a wide spectrum of health benefits, including antibacterial effects, which help prevent infection. Lactoferrin promotes growth, which has implications for human health, particularly for children. I find combinations of soy and whey very attractive, and these are available in excellent nutritional dietary supplement formats created by David Jenkins at Next Nutrition in Carlsbad, California.

It is important to point out that milk protein is not all bad, and some soy milk manufacturers have produced beverages that contain a mixture of both soy and dairy milk, attempting to offer the advantages of both types of protein in one product. For example, in South Korea, a product called Vegemil Youth, developed by Dr. Chai-Won Chung (the owner of Dr. Chung's Soy Food Co., Ltd.) has enjoyed great success and acceptance among the Korean population. It is marketed for consumption by older children and adolescents. This product represents an important development for the soy and dairy industries because the debate about soy and dairy is not always an either/or issue.

Important at all stages of life is the fact that cow's milk promotes superior calcium absorption, but soy milk can overcome this disadvantage when it is fortified with calcium and vitamin D. Another proposed disadvantage of soy milk is the presence of compounds, known as trypsin inhibitors, that inhibit the production of certain enzymes. However, rather than having a negative impact on health, these trypsin inhibitors appear to play a role in preventing colon, breast, and oral cancers. I believe that their positive role in health far outweighs their antinutrient capability.

The Special Role of Phytochemicals

The presence of saponins in soy milk is intriguing. Saponins may have potential to reduce blood cholesterol and inhibit the formation of cancer. These phytochemicals may also have a role in weight reduction and, although as yet not well-defined, have an anti-aging effect.

In addition, there is a possibility that saponins may interfere with the proliferation of HIV virus, which causes AIDS. Individuals with AIDS face many difficulties, one of which is the potential for opportunistic infections of the bowel and poor absorption of food, which leads to "wasting"—that is, weight loss and resulting weakness. In my own clinical experience, such patients are better able to tolerate soy milk than cow's milk. Other anecdotal reports corroborate my observations, and it appears that fermented soy beverages offer definite benefits for AIDS patients who suffer from nutritional disability and gastrointestinal disorders. The AIDS patient may be afforded relief and advantages from soy milk and soy supplements.

Autoimmune Disorders and Cow's Milk

Autoimmune reactions are at the root of many debilitating diseases that are, unfortunately, difficult to treat when they develop. You have probably heard the term "autoimmune" defined as a situation in which the immune system reacts against itself, or turns on itself. What this means is that the body's defense mechanisms, its immune function, attack tissues in the body.

Modern research increasingly indicates that certain foods in the diet may trigger autoimmune responses. It is possible that autoimmunity may be the cause of several common diseases, including Type 1 diabetes mellitus, systemic lupus erythematosus (SLE), and connective tissue diseases such as rheumatoid arthritis.

Some animal studies support the suggestion that the proteins in cow's milk may trigger Type 1 diabetes, and components of whey protein may be responsible for the effect. Researchers claim to have found one of the offending agents in milk, a substance called ABBOS. Through a complex biochemical process, ABBOS can destroy the cells in the pancreas that secrete insulin, thereby triggering Type 1 diabetes mellitus, commonly called juvenile diabetes because it generally affects young people. This type of diabetes is invariably insulin dependent.

Cow's milk has also been implicated as a possible cause of rheumatoid arthritis, inflammatory bowel disease, and systemic lupus erythematosus. Research reports suggest that some patients with rheumatoid arthritis have high levels of antibodies to cow's milk proteins. Certain types of cow's milk protein can cause lesions in rabbits that resemble the tissue changes found with rheumatoid arthritis. Opponents of this theory argue that it has not been clearly demonstrated that cow's milk protein can induce arthritis in humans. However, the findings have been strong enough that some nutritionists advise their rheumatoid arthritis patients to limit their intake of dairy products.

Inflammatory bowel disease is often due to ulcerative colitis or Crohn's disease of the bowel. These disorders have significant associations with autoimmune reactions. Several studies have shown that individuals with inflammatory bowel disease do better when milk protein is eliminated from the diet. Furthermore, individuals with inflammatory bowel disease are universally lactase deficient, and their bowel symptoms become worse when they eat dairy foods.

Based on animal studies, it has been suggested that soy foods may have some potential to cause diabetes. However, overall, there is no evidence that soy foods promote autoimmune disease.

Soy Infant Formula

It goes without saying that breast milk is the standard against which infant formulas are measured, regardless of whether they are based on cow's milk or soy. It was this ideal that Dr. Chai-Won Chung followed with his infant formula Vegemil, which he developed over several decades and extensively tested. It is balanced with the major essential nutrients, nineteen amino acids, twelve vitamins, and twelve minerals. The naturally occurring nutrients in soy, including the oligosaccarhides, fiber, lecithin, saponins, protease inhibitors, and phytonutrients, are included. Over several decades, babies fed with Dr. Chung's soy-based infant formulas have thrived. In fact, he has not received any reports of adverse effects from his formulas.

There have been questions raised about the effects of phytoestrogens in soy formula. Some speculate that the weak estrogenic effect of soy isoflavones, which have caused some fertility problems in animals, could have an adverse effect on human infants. Various speculative reports have fueled a media controversy. However, based on observations of Asian populations, which eat large quantities of soy, this concern appears to be unfounded.

It is important to remember that in response to this controversy, the U.S. Food and Drug Administration and the United Kingdom Department of Health have issued advisories that attest to the safety of soy formulas.

For the most part, soy formula has been viewed as a substitute for cow's milk formula. In other words, if an infant is unable to tolerate cow's milk due to milk allergy or lactose intolerance, then soy-based formulas are used. However, given the extensive experience with soy-based formulas in Asia, the idea that soy is merely a substitute may be too limited. One important difference between the two is that the fat content of soy is of a more health-ful variety than cow's milk, which is high in saturated fat. Soy instead contains health-giving omega-6 and omega-3 fatty acids, no small consideration when one considers the overall health benefits of soy. I regard Dr. Chung as the world expert on infant formulas made with soy, and he is convinced that the isoflavones and omega-3 fatty acids in soy milk afford great advantages. The fatty acid DHA, when given to children, has positive effects on development and I.Q.

A CAUTIONARY NOTE

Soy-based beverages, such as the soy milk sold in supermarkets and health food stores, are not the same as soy infant formulas. True infant formulas are nutritionally complete and designed to nutritionally resemble breast milk. Just as you would not open a carton of milk and feed it to your infant, soy milk should not be used in this manner either.

That said, special soy-based formulas are approved for infant feeding, and should not be considered a second best formula. For children and adults alike, soy-based beverages are a nutritionally attractive alternative to dairy milk. For the lactose intolerant, soy beverages add a varied and healthful drink to their diet. For the AIDS patient, I think they are a godsend.

CHAPTER 13

Soy and the Special Needs of Active Adults and Athletes

This chapter is written for everyone, with my hope that *all* adults recognize that exercise is mandatory for health. A sedentary way of life results in premature death and contributes significantly to chronic degenerative diseases that destroy quality of life, especially in later years. If you have not done so already, I urge you to make a commitment to an exercise program. Ultimately, your health depends on it.

We can learn much about nutrition and its interaction with exercise in promoting health by studying the needs of elite athletes. Finding the optimal diet to meet their nutritional requirements is always a concern for athletes. The goal of this chapter is to provide information about the role of soy in a nutritionally sound program for both athletes and active adults.

EXERCISE AND NUTRITIONAL NEEDS

In a healthy human body, muscle mass accounts for about 40 percent of total body weight. If you want to maintain your youth and achieve optimal health, you have to give this muscle mass regular exercise. One popular way to do it is with aerobic exercise, which includes activities such as running, jogging, walking, stair-climbing, swimming, and sports such as basketball and tennis. In the past few decades, floor and step aerobics have become particularly popular with many women, and the market for aerobic exercise video tapes of all types continues to grow. When we engage in aerobic exercise, oxygen is delivered to the body's tissues and glucose or breakdown products of fats are used to meet energy demands. One of the most important effects of aerobic exercise is that it promotes cardiovascular fitness.

Weight training and toning exercises can be predominately anaerobic exercises, meaning that the tissues are not oxygenated during the exercise. In the absence of oxygenation, acidic metabolites can build up in tissues and decrease the efficiency of muscle function. This is not to say that anaerobic exercises are not valuable. Weight training helps build muscle strength and mass, and many individuals combine aerobic activity with some form of toning or strength-training work. Stretching exercises, yoga, T'ai Chi, and the martial arts increase flexibility and promote a supple body. When performed appropriately, all types of exercise build health.

Muscle tissue requires a readily available source of calories. Body stores of glycogen produce about 50 percent of the energy requirements for exercise, but these stores are usually exhausted within about two hours of continuous activity. The body then draws on fat as an energy source, and fatty acids are burned as fuel. However, to be used efficiently by the body, fatty acids require glucose. When glucose levels fall, performance deteriorates and exhaustion can rapidly set in.

For the average man or woman who engages in thirty- to sixty-minute aerobic activity sessions four or five times a week, exhaustion is not an issue if the diet generally supplies adequate protein, carbohydrates, and fats. It should be noted that the usual nutritional recommendations do not apply at the extremes of indulgence, or lack of indulgence, in exercise. Individuals training for marathons, for example, must prepare for long periods of continuous activity. The more active athlete requires a higher percentage of carbohydrates in the diet than the nonathlete. A minimum of 55 percent of an athlete's daily diet should be comprised of carbohydrates; 70 percent may be the optimal amount for some athletes.

It is important to remember that all carbohydrates are not created equal. Glazed donuts and chocolate cake, for instance, contain primarily simple sugars—along with a considerable amount of fat. Athletes should attempt to derive about 85 percent of all consumed complex carbohydrates in their diets from plant sources. Ideal foods include vegetables, cereals, and legumes such as soy. Traditional soy-based diets are often largely vegetarian and, by definition, rich in complex carbohydrates. I believe that soy foods and soy-based food supplements are ideal for athletes.

The emphasis on lowering fat intake has led some athletes to conclude that they should avoid fats as much as possible. However, fats are necessary to supply essential fatty acids and are a natural source of the fat-soluble vitamins A, D, E, and K. Fats should comprise about 20 percent of the total diet, but we have to consider the factor of "good" fat and "bad" fat in the foods we consume.

Understanding Fats in the Diet

Like carbohydrates, fats can be the basis of fuel for the body. Fats contain elements of carbon, hydrogen, and oxygen, but the ratio of hydrogen to oxygen can vary, which determines the saturation or nonsaturation of fats. Generally speaking, saturated fat is bad fat; it most often is from animal origin and goes with unwanted cholesterol in the diet. Unsaturated fats are generally healthy and are most often of plant origin.

The most important types of health-giving fats are so-called monounsaturated fats and essential fats. Soybeans are a rich source of unsaturated fats and precursors of essential fats of the omega-6 and omega-3 series. Omega-3 type fats are most often found in fish and marine mammals, and they have enormous and versatile health-giving potential. Modern research shows us that omega-3 types of essential fatty acids are important in maintaining cardiovascular, brain, and nerve tissue, as well as skeletal health. The soybean is almost unique in the plant kingdom in containing omega-3 fatty acid precursors, just like fish and marine mammals do.

Fats are a very efficient source of calories, and they are therefore an enemy of the individual who is committed to weight control. Because they have a relatively low oxygen content, fats produce about two-and-one half times the calories found in carbohydrates on a weight-for-weight basis. Some fats are relatively inefficient sources of energy for the sporting enthusiast because they require a greater supply of oxygen than carbohydrates do during their use as fuel in the body's metabolic processes.

Fat is, however, the greatest store of energy in the body. An average young adult is composed of 16-20 percent fat (this varies between males and females), which has a potential energy yield of greater than 120,000 calories. Thus, the average stores of fat in a healthy young adult are enough to provide an inactive person with an adequate supply of calories for three or four months. You can imagine the situation for a person who is well above ideal body weight, and inactive.

In general, individuals eating a Western diet consume at least 50 percent more fat than they may actually require. When the fat is predominately of the saturated type of animal origin, this situation has a detrimental effect on health. Excessive animal fat goes along with excessive animal protein and excessive cholesterol, with their known adverse effects on health and well-being.

The Protein Question

One of the biggest arguments in sports medicine involves the definition of the source and optimal intake of protein in the diet. Protein requirements for athletes always receive considerable attention, and opinions differ widely on the amount of protein needed.

Protein is associated with building and maintaining important structures in the body, and it can be an energy source for
muscle function, although it is a much less efficient energy source
than carbohydrates or fat. It has generally been proposed that the
average adult woman needs about 50 grams of protein a day; the
average adult man needs about 65 grams. Most Westerners have
no difficulty obtaining these amounts—and more. Many
Americans consume about 150 grams of protein a day, which is
not only wasteful (economically and environmentally), but it is
known to contribute to health problems as well. Excess protein
consumption is stressful to the kidneys, and when protein is
derived from animal sources, saturated fat intake is invariably too
high. This high animal protein diet is an important factor in the
cause of coronary artery disease.

Some athletes increase protein intake to up to five times the
normal requirement. This may appear to be a misguided practice,
but athletes do this because they believe extra protein may enhance
their performance, build healthier body structures, increase muscle bulk and strength, or decrease the time it takes to recover from
periods of strenuous activity. Evidence exists showing that athletes
engaged in endurance or power activities may need more protein
than other adults. Some experts propose that an athlete's protein
needs may range from 0.45 to 0.73 grams of protein per pound of
body weight. However, there is no consensus answer to the protein
question.

SCHWARZENEGGER SPEAKS: MUSCULAR ACTIVITY AND PROTEIN

Famous actor and former bodybuilder Arnold Schwarzenegger
has made some extremely insightful comments about protein
needs in his 1981 book, *Arnold's Bodybuilding for Men*. In the
book, Schwarzenegger discusses the use of diets that contain 50 to
70 percent protein, and he describes this approach as "overboard"
and "totally unnecessary." Schwarzenegger advocates consuming
about one gram of protein for every two pounds of body weight.

This level of protein intake is possible with most balanced diets and could be readily achieved with a complete vegetarian approach.

MUSCULAR ACTIVITY AND PROTEIN

There are many studies that clearly show that the combustion of protein in the body is not much higher even during heavy exercise than it is during normal daily routines. Vegetable sources of protein, such as soy, are ideal. They do not have the encumbrances that come with saturated fat, such as cholesterol, fiber deficiency, and simple sugars. The need for protein is directly related to lean body mass. Thus, recommendations of protein intake are best given in grams per kilogram of body weight.

In the early part of this decade, the U.S. FDA recommended a new way of assessing the quality of protein using a tandard called the protein digestibility corrected amino acid score, or PDCAAS for short. Under this now internationally recognized measure of protein quality, soy protein has a PDCAAS score of one, which is equivalent to that of animal, egg, or milk protein.

THE ALLEGED DEFICIENCIES OF SOY PROTEIN ARE REALLY AN ADVANTAGE

I do not stand alone in my strong opinion that soy protein is an ideal protein, even though it is known to have a lower content of the important amino acid methionine. In their book, *The Simple Soybean and Your Health*, Mark and Virginia Messina point out that there is no need to consider improving the quality of soy protein by adding methionine because the lack of methionine becomes a problem only if total protein intake in the diet of an adult is low. Of course, total protein in most Western diets is too high, not too low.

The situation is different for infants who are fed soy formulas. In these foods, methionine is supplemented because a baby's growth requirements demand ubiquitous amino acids. Soy infant formulas have become very popular in many countries because they can be relied upon as a good source of nutrition in circumstances where milk proteins cannot be given. Some scientists with vast clinical and research experience, such as pediatrician Dr. Chai-Won Chung, have gone so far as to recommend soy infant formulas over milk-based infant formulas, and many other physicians have followed suit.

The lack of methionine has been used as a basis to criticize soy, but this characteristic of soy is believed to be one of the reasons that soy protein is so healthful. The amino acid profile of soy, with its low methionine content, helps explain why soy protein can protect against or be beneficial in the prevention of cancer, osteoporosis, cardiovascular disease, and hypertension. Mark Messina has stated, "It may turn out that soy protein is best just as it is."

Excessive protein in the diet cannot be stored by the body. Instead it is broken down and used by the body as a relatively inefficient energy source, or is stored as fat, not as muscle tissue. In other words, increasing protein intake does not in itself lead to a more athletic body. In general, nutritionists recommend a diet in which about 15 percent of total calories derive from protein sources. Athletes generally exceed this recommendation.

Soy Protein is Efficiently Used

There are several reasons why soy protein is desirable for athletes—or for any healthy person. The recommended dietary allowance (RDA) of protein is no doubt a familiar concept, but it is also somewhat misleading. The requirement is actually for amino acids, which are the building blocks of protein structures and the form in which protein takes part in metabolism, the continuous process involving both the breakdown and buildup of the body's energy-producing components. Products of this metabolic process—or recycling—are lost in the body's secretions and excretions, and these losses are replenished by protein consumption in the diet.

TABLE 12
PROTEIN DIGESTIBILITY CORRECTED AMINO ACID
SCORES FOR SELECT FOODS

Product	PDCAAS Score
Genista (soya protein)	1.00
Casein	1.00
Egg White	1.00
Pea Flour	0.69
Pinto beans (canned)	0.63
Kidney beans (canned)	0.68
Lentils (canned)	0.52
Peanut meal	0.52
Rolled oats	0.57
Whole wheat	0.40
Wheat gluten	0.25

Soy protein's advantage in this process is proven in ongoing studies of Olympic athletes in Romania and China. These athletes were given an increased intake of soy protein. When their urine was analyzed it showed a decrease in mucoprotein, a persuasive indication that the soy protein was very efficiently metabolized in their bodies. The athletes' liver and kidney functions remained normal during these tests, and objective measures of their fatigue actually improved.

BUILDING MUSCLE TISSUE

All athletes understand the importance of building muscle tissue to increase strength. To most people, this means less attempting to "sculpt" a body-builder physique than it means achieving an optimal weight, with a healthy ratio of muscle to body fat. Athletes are more health-conscious than ever before, and their knowledge of nutrition is generally quite sophisticated. They routinely look for natural protein formulas for nutritional support in building muscle mass.

Of the numerous muscle-building formulas available, many use soy protein as a base. Many of these formulas come in the form of a kit, which lays out a program of workout regimens, nutritional requirements, and nutrient supplements. Protein is regarded by many trainers as the most important single factor for success in building muscle, and athletes have many choices about the way they will consume protein. I believe that vegetable protein, particularly soy protein, is the healthiest option. Soy protein can efficiently lower cholesterol, may play a role in preventing certain cancers, and promotes healthy digestion. It is important to repeat this information in order to gain a thorough understanding of the real importance soy protein can have for either athlete or active adult. You are advised to buy soy supplements for sports nutrition from companies that lead the field in research and development. The two notable examples are Weider Nutritional International of Salt Lake City, Utah, and Next Nutrition of Carlsbad, California.

MODERN STUDIES SHOW UNEQUIVOCAL BENEFITS OF SOY

Several studies have confirmed benefits from adding soy protein to the diets of elite athletes. Professor I. Dragan of the Institute of Sports Medicine in Bucharest, Romania, has documented that soy protein supplementation during intense training periods results in an increase in lean body mass, a decrease of body fat, and an increase in hemoglobin (the pigment in the circulating red blood cells that carries oxygen) and serum protein concentrations. Soy in the diet has been reported to result in a decrease in fatigue following exercise. Professor Dragan also noted a decrease in secretion of urinary mucoproteins and glycoproteins, which he considered to be indicative of the decrease in the overall stress on the kidneys that occurs with high levels of soy protein supplementation. This distinguished scientist recommends soy supplementation for endurance athletes, and he extended his recommendations recently when he demonstrated beneficial effects of soy protein supplementation for female swimmers.

Professor Huang Quang Min has obtained similar results in a study of forty-two athletes who are members of several Chinese athletic teams. Professor Huang has made several observations. In addition to a reduction in body fat, there was also a reduction in blood viscosity, which means that the blood flowed easily to the small blood vessels. Increases in circulating and cardiac function were additional benefits. This scientist also reported enhanced performance among gymnasts, weightlifters, and members of the badminton team.

Soy Skeptics Are Often Misguided

Trainers and nutritionists who are skeptical about soy express concern about the "estrogenic" effects of isoflavones. However, this concern is unsupported by any facts. Simply no evidence exists for any negative or adverse consequences from the estrogenic components in soy, whether it is consumed as part of a regular diet or taken as a nutritional supplement. The reason for this probably can be traced to the way that soy isoflavones function as adaptogens, so that they end up being antiestrogenic as often as they are proestrogenic.

Fads, Fallacies and Facts

An ongoing criticism leveled at the manufacturers of sports nutrition products is that they "cash in" on fads and fallacies and take advantage of athletes who constantly look for the winning edge. I find, on the contrary, that many manufacturers of these products have expended a great deal of time and money in studying the application of good nutritional principles to athletic activities. Among the leaders in the field is Weider Nutrition International, Inc., which has formulated a high-technology, quality line of soy-based supplements that can be used by active adults and athletes.

In his excellent book, *Diet and Sport*, Wilf Paish talks about the unhealthy obsession that athletes have with drinking milk.

He describes athletes that drink up to ten pints (six liters) of milk per day, based on the misguided notion that milk is one of the most complete foods. Milk is a good food when used in moderation, but it has no advantages to offer over soy milk and has the added disadvantage of presenting a high load of cholesterol and saturated fat.

Soy Shakes

Dairy products and milk often can be replaced by soy foods such as soy milk, tofu, and soy protein, or other soy fractions used as dietary supplements. The U.S. has become a nation of milkshake—or other types of shake—drinkers. Various types of soy protein are the perfect base ingredient for these drinks. Using soy protein in a variety of formats, it is possible to make a concentrated powder that can be mixed with water, juice, or soy milk and has a taste and consistency indistinguishable from common dairy milkshakes. In contrast to standard milkshakes, these soy beverages are delicious, low in calories, and contain no cholesterol or fat.

MUHAMMAD ALI: THE GREATEST OF ALL TIME

In 1996 I had the privilege of spending a few days with Muhammad Ali at his home in Michigan. He would not mind that I tell you about his great passion for milkshakes. Muhammad Ali and his wife Lonnie have been very interested in the health-giving benefits of soy foods, and Ali has endorsed a soyburger made by VitaPro, a company in Montreal, Canada. Both Muhammad and Lonnie were delighted with the chocolate shake I formulated from soy protein, which met some of Ali's special needs and pleased his palate at the same time.

Several companies have entered the field of making soy protein isolates in forms that are readily incorporated into pleasant beverages. Notable among the industry leaders are Protein Technologies, Inc., and the food giant Archer Daniels Midland Corporation. The research departments at these two companies have led the way in supplying the food industry with new formulations for soy-containing foods that promote health and well-being.

Adding Soy Protein

For athletes soy protein isolates, usually in the form of powdered drink mixes, serve as either meal replacements or as supplements to meals. Soy protein also tends to be filling, and foods that promote satiety are advantageous for weight control. Using soy drink mixes to replace some meals is probably safe, but I do not recommend using these drinks to comprise a total weight loss diet.

Soy protein drink mixes are generally bland and therefore take on the flavor of the liquid with which they are blended. This adds to their versatility and practicality. Product labels disclose the percentage of soy protein and the amino acid content, and they will also make you aware of the presence of dairy proteins. Given the range of products, it pays to read the label carefully. Some natural food markets and fitness stores carry soy protein powders as one component of a program designed for athletes, or for active adults who engage in strenuous aerobic or weight-training activities. To maximize results, I recommend working with a knowledgeable athletic trainer or a health-care professional who can tailor a supplementation program that meets your specific needs.

EXAMINING THE TYPES OF SOY DIETARY AND NUTRITIONAL SUPPLEMENTS

It is clear that soy is versatile as a basis for making many different types of supplements for either an athlete or a healthy adult. Soy protein powders can be taken "straight" in liquid form, added to beverages, prepared as premixed beverages, mixed with food, and even made into candy bars. In a recent sports nutrition field study, I created a line of dietary supplements called Team Choice in collaboration with several professional athletes, trainers, and even referees.

In this project, the Team Choice line had to fulfill the criteria of being able to provide necessary nutritional needs such as protein and energy; be in a convenient, palatable format; and, of course, have major health-promoting abilities. In the initial study of the Team Choice line, soy beverage was placed in a field study research program with Mark Letendre, head trainer of the San Francisco Giants; Herm Schneider, head trainer of the Chicago White Sox; and Sandy Alomar, the acclaimed superstar catcher for the Cleveland Indians. Suffice it to say that soy made the task of creating this line easy. The Team Choice energizing beverages with soy protein and carbohydrate loading proved highly acceptable and effective when used by trainers and professional athletes. Weider Nutritional International has formulated some exciting new soy powder mixes for athletes, which contain healthful amounts of isoflavones.

EXERCISE AND HEALTH

In my book on lifestyle published by Keats, I stress the importance of exercise as a lifestyle adjustment that makes very important contributions to physical and mental well-being. There are many misconceptions about the role of exercise in health promotion. For one thing, it is not necessary to imitate the athlete who trains arduously for competition. Typical adult fitness buffs are not preparing themselves for competitive events—they compete with themselves, and so their motivation comes from within.

Exercise has a very beneficial effect on the heart, lungs, muscles, joints, and bones. After exercise is sustained for as little as fifteen minutes, notable improvements can be measured in tests of cardiovascular and respiratory function. It is never too early or too late in life to exercise. Mature adults may wish to take it easy at the start and are advised to seek the guidance of a trainer or physician if any health concerns exist.

DIETARY SUPPLEMENTS

It is frequently stated that if one eats a balanced diet, then vitamin, mineral, or herbal supplements are not necessary. This short-sighted viewpoint assumes that it is easy to eat a balanced diet—which is not true—and that the majority of readily available food is nutritious, which is also not true. The lifestyle of the more physically active person differs fundamentally from most people. It could be assumed that they have adopted a more disciplined routine in their lives than most other people. However, just like the committed athlete, the busy nonathlete is short on time and does not often relax over a satisfying meal. Small wonder that such individuals recognize the need to supplement their diets with well-selected dietary supplements, or so-called "nutriceuticals." Unfortunately, the availability and abundance of these supplements often is not supported by a source of sound, practical advice.

Some authors dismiss the need for carbohydrate and fat "therapy," somewhat ill-advisedly, in my opinion. Carbohy-drate intake in the diet of the active adult should be sufficient to promote readily assimilable energy, and it is more healthy if it is taken in the form of complex sugars that come with a good dose of health-giving dietary fiber. The role of essential fatty acids, especially of the omega-3 type, which is found in fish oil, has also in the past been underestimated in its importance for promoting cardiovascular, skeletal, and nervous system health. Protein therapy is favored by many trainers and athletes, and we have reviewed the advantages of soy and vegetable protein sources, which are available as supplements or in soy foods. Some athletes and trainers supplement amino acids, which are known to have effects on hormones (growth hormone, glucagon, and insulin), and can affect muscle growth and other body functions. However, for most people supplementing the diet with expensive concoctions of amino acids (*e.g.*, arginine and ornithine) has little advantage to offer over good, balanced protein intake that is in a readily digestible form.

Digestibility of food is a very important issue for the adult involved in a regular exercise program. High-energy density foods (high caloric content per volume) are good at promoting satiety, but they hang around in the digestive tract and draw blood flow to the gut area, away from other vital organs during exercise—if such foods are eaten prior to exercise. Most soy foods contain easily digestible carbohydrates, protein, and fat content. Mark Messina has pointed out that soy protein isolates are approximately 95 percent digestible, and tofu is greater than 90 percent digested.

PLEASE DO NOT MESS WITH YOUR BODY!

Many trainers and sports experts report favorable outcomes with the use of vitamin and mineral supplements, when used appropriately. Colloidal minerals, prepared in microscopically small particles, are often considered gimmicks, and their safety has been questioned. Pollen extracts have met with variable success, but cruciferous greens seem to hold promise for providing a health-giving array of vitamins, minerals, and essential nutrients. A very successful product in this area is Emerald Greens, a special formulation of vegetable components, including soy. Emerald Greens was developed by the world-famous naturopath, Dr. Tony O'Donnell from Ireland, via Los Angeles, California.

A word of caution may be tiresome to some athletes, but I still want to add that messing around with anabolic steroids, stimulant drugs, and unproven herbal concoctions is just not worth the risk. There has also been major interest in the use of DHEA (dehydroepiandrosterone), a hormone precursor, but before supplementing with DHEA I advise athletes and active adults to check with a health-care professional. Soy isoflavones have "bothered" some male athletes, but few body builders need more androgens. Remember, soy isoflavones are adaptogens, not just estrogens.

PHYSICAL FITNESS SAVES LIVES

A person's state of physical fitness is often associated with mental well-being and a greater resistance to disease. Physical fitness is such an important predictor for mortality that it behooves all of us to try to exercise regularly. Researchers at institutions such as Harvard Medical School in Boston, Massachusetts, are reporting excellent results for enhancement of physical and emotional well-being in the elderly by the application of fairly simple, but sustained, exercise programs.

Good nutrition and regular exercise are two lifestyle adjustments that are well within the reach of the average person. You supply the exercise, and soy—with its great health-giving qualities—can supply an important part of the nutrition.

CHAPTER 14

Soy and Your Children

Our society is in the midst of a transition about the role of diet in preventing the life-threatening diseases discussed in this book. Two fundamental components of our diet—dairy products and animal protein—are under increasing scrutiny. Health-conscious adults have been learning more about a healthful diet for several decades, but many are still confused about what is best for their children.

In a society whose health-care establishment has traditionally focused on treatment rather than prevention, discussions about adequate diets for children take on a casual tone. The attitude appears to go something like this: As long as children drink *enough* milk and eat *enough* protein to promote growth, then it does not matter all that much what else they eat. At some point in the future, usually after they are adults, medical tests may reveal high cholesterol levels, elevated blood pressure, signs of diabetes, and so forth, and at that point, they can become concerned about their diet or so the attribute goes. This casual attitude often prevails into early adulthood, and even beyond, if no measurable or visible signs of ill health appear. Many adults simply are not aware that these adult diseases may not have developed in the first place had the childhood diet been focused on long-term health and prevention.

Sometimes the most well-intentioned parents will decide that changing their children's diet is too difficult and may not even be wise. They do not want their children to be different from their neighbors' children, or the pressure to take their kids to fast-food places—as well as the convenience—is too great to resist. Besides, their doctor or grandparents may tell them the children are healthy and not to worry so much. These pressures are real. Deciding that milkshakes, cheeseburgers, and french fries are not good for your child may pit your will against your child, your child's school, and perhaps even your pediatrician or family physician.

Given that fast food is relatively inexpensive and unarguably convenient, it is also understandable that many working parents use these restaurants as a substitute for the tedious task of cooking at home every day. Overworked and tired parents are not figments of the imagination, and I do not discount these issues.

Unfortunately, however, many parents are unaware of the consequences of a high-fat diet in childhood.

SIGNS OF EARLY DAMAGE

Evidence that heart disease begins early appeared decades ago in the reports of autopsies performed on young soldiers killed during the Korean and Vietnam conflicts. These men were generally between the ages of twenty and twenty-two and presumed to be healthy when they entered military service. However, 70 percent of the U.S soldiers showed signs of coronary artery disease. Of note, however, is that the young Asian soldiers who died in these conflicts did not show similar signs. Since cardiovascular disease takes years to develop, it is almost certain that the damage to the U.S. soldiers began in childhood. While stress contributes to heart disease, it is unlikely that the temporary psychological pressure of war-time conditions was the cause of early coronary artery disease, particularly because Asian soldiers, who were subjected to the same stress, often had smooth, undamaged arteries.

By now you will not be surprised that I point to the plant-based diet of Asian populations as an explanation for the difference in the health status of these young men at the time of their death. The war-time data are not all we have to go on, however. The same signs of early cardiovascular disease also have been observed during the autopsies of young accident victims in the United States. Yet, despite this data, little has been done to warn parents that their children are at risk when the majority of their diet is comprised of high-fat, animal-protein based foods. Children in Western societies tend to consume most of their fat from meat and dairy products as well as from some highly saturated fats that are used in commercial food processing. Parents who are concerned about their children's consumption of food high in cholesterol are forgetting that the amount of saturated fat in the diet is at least as important as total cholesterol. The young U.S. soldiers did not have coronary artery damage just because they ate meat, but rather because their total diet was unbalanced, with fat comprising a large percentage of calories consumed. Children in rural Japan and China usually consume a diet in which about 10 percent of their total calories come from fat sources. Children in the United States typically consume 40 to 50 percent of their calories from saturated fat sources.

Typically, Westerners believe that their privileged children are the most well-fed young people in the world. They have assumed that the obvious abundance of food means that the nutritional value of the food also must be high. In addition, of course, we have all viewed television images of starving children in countries plagued by natural disasters or military conflict. These tragedies reinforce the notion that Western children must be very healthy indeed because most have never been undernourished. There is no question that the average child in the U.S. consumes adequate calories, but the source of those calories may not promote optimal health. In fact, the rise of obesity in young people speaks volumes about the mistake of confusing quantity with quality. The most common nutritional problem in Western society is overnutrition, not undernutrition. Overnutrition must be perceived as a common form of malnutrition.

Chubby is Not Healthy

Twenty-five percent of children in the United States are over-weight. Over the past several decades, a number of forces have converged to produce heavier children—and heavier adults. The relative sedentary lifestyle of today's children is certainly a factor. Few children walk to school, and the average school-age child watches about five hours of television a day and may spend many more hours engaged in playing video games—or even surfing the Internet. If these young people exercise at all, it is generally while participating in an organized team sport.

It is no coincidence that commercials featuring high-fat foods comprise over 40 percent of the commercials shown during Saturday morning television hours, a time when millions of children are watching. In addition, many children eat breakfast and lunch in school, and much of the food served is high in total fat. For decades now, the beef and dairy industries have conducted intense lobbying to ensure that cheese, hamburger, whole milk, puddings, ice cream, and so forth are considered essential for nutritionally balanced meals served in schools. Many parents are convinced that these foods are the best sources of protein and other nutrients, particularly calcium. Without the support of an informed family physician or pediatrician, it is difficult to buck this system. People who have gone against the fast-food industry have experienced their wrath and unlimited power.

Children Do Not Always Shed Their "Baby" Fat

The folklore of obesity assures us that children will simply out-grow their childhood chubbiness. However, statistics show that this is wishful thinking. The cruelty here is that overweight children suffer ridicule from their peers and mixed messages from adults. Eventually the "cuteness" of baby fat turns into the stigma of being an overweight child, and suddenly the parents are concerned and begin to fuss over the child's eating habits. Since about

25 percent of adults are overweight, the problem obviously is not one that is easily outgrown. According to a 1994 report issued by the Centers for Disease Control, adults between the ages of twenty-five and thirty are, on average, ten pounds heavier than they were even seven years earlier. The rise of childhood obesity is obviously carrying over to adulthood.

Given what we know about the early appearance of heart disease and the health risks that obesity poses, it is time that parents created a diet revolution of their own. This will not be easy because, in some ways, our society may actually be in a period of regression in its concern about healthful eating. A recent consumer research report, presented to the American Dietetic Association's annual meeting in Boston in 1997, stated that only 28 percent of homemakers claim to be cautious about the calorie content of the food they serve at home. This figure was down from almost 39 percent of homemakers who, in a 1990 survey, said they were concerned about calories. Only 43 percent of those surveyed said that it was important to be cautious about the fat content of food; again, this is down from 51 percent in 1990.

Quite properly, this information raises concerns about changing attitudes among U.S. consumers. With all the media reports over the last two decades about the need to lower fat and add more grains and vegetables to the diet, many consumers do not see drastic changes in the health status of their peers. Parents may wonder if it is worth it to put in the effort to change their own eating habits, let alone their children's diet.

IS A DESIRE FOR FAT NATURAL?

Many parents believe their children love fatty foods because it is natural to prefer them over grains or fruits and vegetables. Conventional wisdom would have you believe that a craving for high-fat foods is in-born, but that we must learn to like vegetables. In our society we treat high-fat, sweet foods as special. Social occasions feature these rich desserts and even toddlers know that cake and ice cream are birthday party foods. Perhaps we keep these foods special, so that while we do not deny children some of these treats, their "specialness" makes them a priority in the daily diet.

Despite the notion that there is both a "fat" tooth and a "sweet" tooth, Western children do not have a special gene that leads them to prefer these foods; no one has taste buds for fat. Children develop a "fat habit" because they are fed high-fat foods. If children are given low-fat foods, they will learn to prefer them. Many children are conditioned to associate desserts and snack foods as a "reward" for eating vegetables or behaving well at Grandma's house or even for achieving good grades. The treat and reward mentality involving food is nearly universal in our culture.

To date, however, the health-care establishment has stopped short of actually recommending that calories derived from fat should comprise less than about 30 percent of the diet. Recommendations to eat reduced or low-fat foods have led consumers to believe that they can make small changes here and there and achieve results. Remember, too, that the type of fat consumed is important. Saturated fat is generally not healthful, while unsaturated fat in moderation is essential for health. Parents are usually advised to watch what their children eat and cut down on snacks and sweet, high-fat food, but fundamental changes generally are not urged. It is no wonder that adults are confused and may believe the whole issue is just so much nonsense. And the growth of the fast-food industry surely has not helped.

For a variety of reasons, most health-care professionals do not recommend that adults or children eat a plant-based diet that includes only small amounts of animal protein, or none at all. They believe this is a compliance issue. If they tell you, for example, that animal protein is neither necessary nor desired, you may stop listening because you cannot imagine a diet in which animal protein does not have a central role. So, instead of telling you the whole story, they try to make dietary changes more palatable. After all, in our culture, vegetarians are still considered somewhat odd. The important point here is that it is possible to move toward a vegetable-based diet while still eating some animal protein. A move toward health should be a pleasant experience, not one filled with family squabbles over food or a constant sense of deprivation because one's favorite foods are taken away.

While it is true that basic dietary changes are difficult, the health benefits are worth making the effort. Children who are raised on soy foods like them, just as most children in the U.S. like hamburger. Children could be encouraged to like soyburgers, just as giving children hamburgers encourages favoring them. In Asian countries, soy is not hidden in food products or made to taste like ham or hot dogs. Our taste is conditioned, and there is simply no reason to continue eating habits that may, in the long run, be detrimental to health.

SOY FOODS ARE VERSATILE AND HEALTHFUL

Soy food products are so widely available today that adding them to your children's diet will not add hours of shopping or even preparation time. Many books are available that include recipes for everything from a breakfast soy milk "smoothie" to a hearty tofu lasagna—even puddings and other sweets are available using soy products as a base.

As you have read in this book, soy protein is a complete protein. All essential amino acids are supplied, and the protein is easily handled by the body. In addition, soybeans are naturally a low-fat food, with an average fat content of about 18 percent.

I do not support basing a child's diet on foods to which soy has been added in great amounts, such as commercial baked goods. Nor do I support frying animal protein in soy oil, which destroys the beneficial properties of the oil. What I suggest is adding soy foods into your child's diet in moderate and sensible ways. Given what you have read thus far in this book, there are so many advantages of vegetable protein-based diets in general, and soy foods in particular, that to exclude them because of their fat content makes no sense. The nutritional profile of soy makes it one of nature's "super foods," and I encourage you to introduce your children to the abundant variety of soy-based foods that are available to Westerners today.

CHAPTER 15

Many Other Health Benefits of Soy

In this chapter, I propose findings in some areas of emerging research that further demonstrate the wide range of disease states that may be tackled to some degree by soy or its constituents. In some examples of the application of soy to specific disease states in this chapter, my comments are more speculative than they may be in other sections of the book. These are emerging areas of research, but I have been careful to attempt to separate fact from supposition. Many readers will find this section thought-provoking, and I hope that some scientists are inspired to do research on some of the unanswered questions.

Soy is emerging as a "star" in preventing the serious, degenerative diseases that plague Western society. However, there are other health issues to address. One particularly intriguing issue is the potential relationship between soy-based diets and longevity.

PREVENTING CHRONIC DISEASES IS THE KEY

If you examine the reasons for most premature morbidity and mortality in Western society, it becomes obvious that common chronic diseases are the problem. These diseases are most often related to lifestyle factors such as diet. Most people live into their seventh decade, but humans have the potential to live for a century. It has been estimated that the elimination of cardiovascular disease, the number one cause of death in the West, could add about six years to an average person's life expectancy. Eliminating cancer, together with the other forms of cardiovascular disease, such as stroke, could add sixteen years of survival, with the average person attaining a life expectancy of a hundred years. It is notable that soy-based diets promote cardiovascular wellness and exert a preventive role against cancer.

Populations identified for their longevity have known characteristics: they tend to consume diets low in animal protein, their fiber intake is high, they offer a social structure that is supportive of its members, and they exercise. Further data gathered from longevity studies reveal that not only are vegetable foods a feature of the lifelong diet of centenarians, but their diet is generally high in nutrients and trace elements and lacks refined sugar or heavily processed food.

A clear link seems to exist between caloric intake and a long life span, with the overall calorie consumption among those who live a long time about one-half that of a typical American diet. Among centenarians, obesity is a rare occurrence; obesity is also uncommon in many Asian countries. According to the head monk of the Temple of the Jade Buddha in Shanghai, longevity among monks is common, and their lifestyle fits the findings of nutritional factors in studies of longevity. Buddhists monks also receive credit for demonstrating the culinary versatility of the soybean and creating soy dishes that resemble in taste foods made from animal protein.

Soybeans are nutritionally "wealthy," and it is their abundance of nutritional factors that makes them an ideal supplement to the diet. For instance, they are rich in antioxidants, which have wide-ranging anti-aging and disease-prevention properties. In one important study, a group of laboratory animals was fed a diet based on soybeans while another group was fed a diet based on casein (milk protein). The group that received soybeans had a significant (13 percent) increase in life span compared with the group fed casein. It has been proposed that the amino acids in soybeans resist oxidation and are less likely to introduce free radicals into the body than other protein sources.

The well-known author and nutrition expert, Earl Mindell, Ph.D., author of *The Vitamin Bible* and *The Herb Bible*, traces his interest in soy-based diets to their role in promoting longevity among certain groups of Japanese people. Certainly, the value of soy in promoting cardiovascular wellness and cancer prevention speaks for itself. Table 1 (in Chapter 1) provides a brief summary of the possible role of soy in promoting longevity. Adding soy to the diet while continuing to consume high-fat, high-calorie processed foods is not the way to increase health or add years to your life. The recommendation for consuming soy foods is based on a sensible lifestyle program with the goal of preventing chronic, degenerative diseases. The important thing to remember is that soy offers a nutritionally superior food that is also nearly universally affordable. Soybeans are one of the least expensive sources of health-building proteins, carbohydrates, and healthy fats, plus nature's most abundant source of versatile isoflavones.

DEVELOPMENTS IN ANTI-AGING MEDICINE

The role of antioxidants in preventing chronic disease and prolonging life expectancy is an area of intense research interest. Soy isoflavones are powerful antioxidants, and some of the major health-giving properties of soy come directly from isoflavones and their antioxidant properties. Groundbreaking studies on the role of the prolongation of lifespan in insects by the use of antioxidants, reported in *Science* in 1994 by Dr. W. C. Orr and Dr. R. S. Sohal, have fueled many recent clinical studies in humans and animals.

Oxidative stress promotes chronic degenerative disease and tissue aging. In particular, it plays a significant role in causing cancer, which is a principal cause of premature death throughout the world. Questions remain about whether or not we are choosing the right antioxidants in the right format, and whether they are hitting the targets in the cells they are supposed to.

WHAT ARE THE RIGHT ANTIOXIDANTS?

A Nobel prize is waiting for the researchers who can answer this question because I believe they will have unlocked the door to move us closer towards health and longevity. There is no question that antioxidants have different potencies in their ability to scavenge free radicals that cause oxidative damage to tissues. This potency is, in simple terms, a function of their REDOX potential (ability to mop up radicals that damage tissues). Several antioxidants will tend to be more soluble in fats than water and vice versa (hydrophilic—*i.e.*, "water loving"—versus hydrophobic or lipophilic, or "fat loving"). Not enough attention has been paid to combining hydrophilic and lipophilic antioxidants together to achieve maximum effect in accessing both the water and fatty components (membranes and organelles) of cells.

The principal issue that is debated is a better way of delivering antioxidants to cells by some form of antioxidant "delivery system." It has been recognized that certain antioxidants, such as the hormone melatonin, can freely access most areas of a cell, but the use of hormones such as melatonin are not without drawbacks. I speculate that one of the intrinsic benefits of soy isoflavones is that they have their own built-in delivery potential because they can freely access receptors within cells, as evidenced by their affinity for estrogen receptors. Thus, I postulate that isoflavones are efficient antioxidants because they have their own special type of delivery mechanism to key sites in the cells.

JAPANESE PEOPLE LIVE LONGER

It is probably naive to explain the longevity of Japanese people solely in terms of their predilection for soy in their diet. Nobody has a clear answer to explain the increased life span enjoyed by some communities in Japan. I believe that soy food does play a role, but other factors such as a low-fat, essential fatty-acid rich, low-cholesterol diet are also present. Population studies in Japan have postulated a relationship between longevity and the consumption of soybeans, buckwheat (*soba*), and millet (*hie* or *awa*) instead of refined white rice.

The link between soybean diets and both cancer prevention and longevity has been explained in terms of the ability of the nondigestible sugars (*e.g.*, raffinose and stachyose) in soybeans to promote the growth of friendly bacteria in the large bowel. Not only do such friendly bacteria (commonly, bifidobacteria) help prevent colon cancer, they may have more far-reaching effects in the body, such as the enhancement of immune function that is known to otherwise decline with age. Perhaps very important is the fact that promoting the growth of bifidobacteria with soy will assist in eradicating yeast from the bowel. Soy could be of benefit in breaking the postulated "yeast connection" of diseases.

The most notable group of long-living individuals in Japan are those who live in rural areas on the islands of Okinawa. These individuals eat generous amounts of green and yellow vegetables, which are abundant in antioxidants, and they have an affinity for soybeans.

Soy is definitely not the whole answer. Green tea has been recognized in Japan as a cancer-preventive agent in the diet. News of its benefit is beginning to spread to health-care givers in many Western countries. The active constituent of green tea that is believed to confer its properties as an anticancer agent is epigallocatechin gallate (EGCg), a condensed tannin or catechin. Catechins are present in many different types of tea, but it is EGCg that appears to be relatively specific as an anticancer agent in humans and animals. Epigallocatechin gallate, like soy isoflavones, is a powerful antioxidant in humans and animals.

SOY AND SKIN DISEASES

Westerners often admire the skin of Asian people because of its lack of blemishes and skin disorders. In fact, dermatology is not a very well-developed medical specialty in southeast Asian countries because many common skin diseases that affect Westerners are quite rare. Acne is conspicuous by its absence in Asia, and common eczema or psoriasis are rare in China and Japan. In Western societies, however, acne is by far the most common skin disease. About 80 percent of the U.S. population may experience episodes of acne in their lifetime, and about 25 percent of this group will need some form of treatment for the disorder.

There are several misconceptions about the cause and treatment of acne. Acne may not be caused by dirt or poor hygiene, stress, sexual activity, or specific foods. Acne treatment is often discussed only from the point of view of precipitation of the disorder without an examination of diet as a preventive measure. In my opinion, the role of soy diets and the potential of soy isoflavones for acne prevention have been overlooked by dermatologists in Western communities.

How Acne Begins

Acne primarily affects the hair follicles and sebaceous glands on the face, chest, and back. The sebaceous glands are responsible for keeping the skin and hair lubricated; sebum is the oily secretion of the sebaceous glands. Sebum flows into the hair follicle and reaches the skin surface via the pilosebaceous duct. It is essentially a blockage of this duct that causes excretions to back up and, together with dead cells, result in blackheads and whiteheads (comedones) and other skin lesions, such as the skin eruptions commonly called pimples and acne cysts.

It is widely recognized that male hormones (androgens) are the only hormones that stimulate the sebaceous glands to enlarge and produce sebum. Acne is a common manifestation when androgens are produced in excess in the body. Estrogens have the ability to block the effects of androgens on the sebaceous glands, with a reduction in the size of the oil (sebaceous) glands and a decrease in the amount of sebum that is excreted. This knowledge explains several important aspects of the cause, treatment, and prevention of acne.

The beneficial effects of estrogen on the course of acne in young females has led to the use of the birth control pill, which contains potent estrogens, in treating unresponsive acne. Obviously, this treatment has limitations. Oral contraceptives have side effects, including nausea, weight gain, breast tenderness, intermenstrual spotting, and the risk of vascular disease. Furthermore, the low-dose contraceptive pill is not effective for treating acne, and obviously, estrogen therapy is not suitable for males.

The isoflavones in soy enter this picture because the weak estrogenic effects of soy isoflavones represent an ideal dietary measure to prevent or control acne. What I propose is that soy isoflavones function as antiandrogens that may assist in blocking the effect of androgens on the sebaceous glands. Certainly enough evidence exists to conduct clinical trials using soy isoflavones as a natural treatment. If a natural therapy is available to treat any disease, including acne, it should be tried. Soy isoflavones have no known side effects, and their cost makes them an economical alternative to other acne treatments.

Does Beautiful Skin Need to Cost a Small Fortune?

Beautiful skin is not beautiful if it displays hair where it is desired. Western women spend small fortunes to remove unwanted body hair. Abrasion techniques, bleaching, waxing, plucking, electrolysis depilation, and shaving are inconvenient and expensive. As millions of women will attest, the whole business of unwanted body hair is one big nuisance. But, women seldom stop to ask why they have the hair in the first place.

Generally speaking, dark-haired women have more difficulties with unwanted body hair than fair-haired women. However, dark-haired eastern Asian women are an exception to this "rule." In general, eastern Asian women living in Asia have far fewer problems with unwanted hair than Western women. I believe this is a function of dietary differences, with soy being the most significant factor.

Excessive body hair in women is associated with androgenic (male) hormone stimulation. It is well recognized that disease states in women that are associated with excessive androgen secretions in the body cause both acne and excessive body hair (hirsutism). The haphazard growth of body hair is so common among Western women that it is considered normal in women after puberty. Asian women, on the other hand, consume isoflavones in their soy-based diets. The result for them is that the estrogenic effects of isoflavones appear to modulate androgenic stimulation, and prevent the growth of unwanted body hair.

Isoflavones can be used therapeutically in the form of supplements, which have the advantage of offering a stable and predictable dose. Adding soy foods to the diet is, of course, another way to consume isoflavones, although the total intake per day is less predictable from food sources than it would be from an isoflavone supplement.

Psoriasis, Eczema, and Angiogenesis

The role of soy-based diets in the prevention of psoriasis or eczema is not as direct as their role in preventing or treating acne. However, I believe that the antiangiogenic effects of soy isoflavones are potentially beneficial in these common skin disorders. Angiogenesis is the growth of new blood vessels; antiangiogenesis inhibits the growth of new blood vessels. Angiogensis is essential for repairing and healing the body. But there are times when it can have a negative effect, as when it increases the inflammation of arthritis or helps cancerous tumors grow, or furthers the symptoms of skin conditions such as psoriasis and eczema. Isoflavones share with shark cartilage the ability to modulate angiogenesis, and therefore help people who suffer with these skin diseases.

Joshua R. Korzenik, M.D., in collaboration with Stephen Barnes, Ph.D., have preliminary results on the use of soy protein containing isoflavones in the treatment of an uncommon condition called hereditary hemorrhagic telangiectasia. This disease runs in families and is characterized by the occurrence of nosebleeds, hemorrhage from the gastrointestinal tract, and the variable occurrence of migraine headache. Individuals with this disorder bleed from the clumps of dilated blood vessels (telangiectasis) that can occur in the mouth, nose, and gut.

This study is an ideal human model in which to study the antiangiogenic effects of isoflavones. Eight of nine patients who took soy protein containing isoflavones in their diet had variable but positive responses to soy. Six of the patients had nose bleeds, and three of these individuals had complete—or near complete—cessation of nasal hemorrhages. One of three of the people with hereditary hemorrhagic telangiectasia had a marked positive response to the soy in the diet, associated with a diminished need for blood transfusions and a partial correction of their severe anemia. It is notable that four patients with migraine had relief of their headaches. Unfortunately, the cause of the headaches in this disease is not completely understood, but this observation may justify the study of isoflavones as an adjunct to the management of the very common and distressing migraine disorder.

The importance of these preliminary observations rests in the fact that soy protein with isoflavones seems to be causing measurable antiangiogenic effects in humans. These are truly exciting observations, and the angio-modulating effects of soy isoflavones in wound healing and tissue repair deserve more study.

ISOFLAVONES AND ALCOHOL ABUSE?

From tests on animals, Dr. Renee C. Lin and Dr. Ting-Kaili from the Department of Medicine and Biochemistry at Indiana University School of Medicine have presented some intriguing findings on the isoflavone daidzein and its effect on alcohol drinking behavior, as well as the degree of inebriation achievable from alcohol intake. These researchers showed that daidzein was able to shorten the sleep time experienced by rats who were fed alcohol directly into their stomach—the sleep time indicating inebriation—while, in separate experiments, daidzein reduced the voluntary drinking of alcohol by rats.

The mechanism of the anti-inebriant and the antidipsotropic (reducing drinking) effects of daidzein are not completely understood, but they have been proposed to be related to the ability of isoflavones to delay the emptying of the stomach. The idea that the soy isoflavones can possibly suppress the appetite for alcohol and lessen the intoxicating effects of alcohol, presumably by effects on the brain, is intriguing. There are many reasons proposed to explain the intolerance to alcohol experienced by Orientals and their low incidence of alcohol abuse. Along with a metabolic intolerance to alcohol that is a genetic feature of Oriental people, could isoflavones in their diet also be protective against excessive alcohol intake?

THE INTRIGUING ISSUE OF SOY AND RADIATION INJURY

It is well-known that environmental factors may cause or promote the growth of cancer. This is never more evident than with the risk of radiation exposure. Two incidents of catastrophic radiation exposure provide information about soy and its potential to protect against radiation-induced injury—the dropping of atomic bombs on Hiroshima and Nagasaki. The bombs killed hundreds of thousands of people, but, equally important, had long-lasting effects on the surviving Japanese population, who suffered the terrible misery of radiation-induced cancers in diverse forms.

In a newspaper article in the *Japan Times*, Dr. Shinichiro Akizuki of Saint Francisco Hospital in Nagasaki, Japan, offered an opinion that one of the reasons that physicians who attended atomic bomb victims did not suffer significant radiation-related illnesses was that they consumed miso, a soybean product. In support of Dr. Akizuki's view, there are animal studies where miso has been shown to reduce radiation-induced neoplasia. It has been shown quite definitively that soy products can reduce the risk of spontaneous and radiation-induced liver tumors in mice. The use of soy protein isolates as dietary supplements to prevent radiation-induced cancer could be a very important potential intervention. As the radiation leak at Chernobyl proved as well as the tension created by nuclear detonations in 1998 by India and Pakistan, there are no ironclad guarantees that we will never have to face this problem on a greater or lesser scale.

CHAPTER 16

Safety and Application of Soy

ADVERSE EFFECTS OF SOY: FACT OR FICTION?

Claims about the "super value" of any food or nutrient is and perhaps should always be met with healthy skepticism. There is nothing inherently wrong with refusing to jump on a dietary or nutritional bandwagon and, in fact, premature endorsement of any medical development often leads to disappointment after all the facts surface. New surgical procedures and drugs frequently are heralded as "miracles," but when failure rates or adverse side effects become known, the miracle does not seem so assured. The same is true for many developments in the world of alternative medicine, too. Nutritional medicine is fraught with myths and magical thinking. Fortunately, pseudoscience in nutrition is being replaced rapidly by logical reasoning, and more research points to the unequivocal benefits of certain types of nutritional intervention.

In my opinion, the benefits of soy do not fit into a scenario of promising more than it can deliver, but it remains difficult to convince many of my colleagues. Soy has been a staple food for billions of people over a period of several thousand years. It is mystifying that the scientific evidence that confirms soy's value in building and maintaining health has been all but ignored for so long. While it is true that it can take time for new foods and dietary concepts to gain acceptance, information about the health benefits of soy have not been widely disseminated in conventional health-care arenas. Western populations have not been encouraged to expand their dietary horizons. In some cases, it would seem that the medical community has resisted the positive information and, instead, have focused on reports of potential adverse effects of soy—reports that are not particularly relevant to humans. I do not wish to delve into the dichotomy of conventional and alternative medicine, but both disciplines have been shortsighted in their use of soy as a health-giving principle in the diet.

THE PHYTOESTROGEN SAGA

One of the most frequent misrepresentations about soy foods concerns the effects of isoflavones—phytoestrogens—on fertility in humans. Most of the evidence about the effects of isoflavones on fertility is forthcoming from observations of animals. The early work on the biological significance of isoflavones was performed by veterinary scientists. Specifically, fertility problems were noted among sheep and cattle that were fed certain forage plants, such as alfalfa and clover, which contain high concentrations of phytoestrogens. It appeared that phytoestrogens interfered with several hormonal mechanisms that affect reproduction. It is interesting that this work, which is decades old, has recently prompted investments by a major pharmaceutical company in acquiring patents on the isolation of hormonal modifying compounds from forage plants.

Despite the implications of these important observations for domestic animals, no similar adverse effect has ever emerged among humans. The Japanese population, for example, relies heavily on soy foods, and their average isoflavone intake is high when compared to Western populations. Yet, the Japanese have no history of fertility difficulties. The same can be said of other Asian populations. The decreasing birth rate in China is unquestionably due to austere government-sponsored family-planning policies, not a soy-based diet!

There are great differences in the way animals and humans metabolize isoflavones. This difference was illustrated by a situation that developed in some zoos in the United States. Cheetah populations in these zoos exhibited poor survival and reproductive capacity, the cause of which was later determined to be their diet of horsemeat and soybeans. These cheetahs were ingesting relatively large amounts of dietary estrogens, including phytoestrogens. In addition to affecting longevity and fertility, the cheetahs developed liver toxicity. The toxicity appears to be related to an inability of cheetahs and other cats to metabolize dietary phytoestrogens; estrogens can build up and cause toxicity in these animals. There is no evidence that humans have a similar problem handling these types of phytoestrogens.

Animal models that are close to humans on the evolutionary scale provide information that must be considered portable to humans. Studies of the metabolic products (compounds produced by the body) of phytoestrogens, such as equol, help us understand differences among species in the metabolism of isoflavones. Urinary equol excretion, which is a measure of phytoestrogen metabolism, can be used as a means of inferring differences in isoflavone metabolism. Information to date suggests that humans are not able to form equol as several animals do, and this type of difference in the handling of phytoestrogens helps to explain the lack of effects of estrogenic compounds, such as isoflavones, on human reproductive function, in comparison to that observed in some species of animals.

Measurement of isoflavonoids in body fluids shows that the highest values are found in the Japanese—people who have a macrobiotic, or soy-based vegetarian diet—and, to a lesser degree, a lactovegetarian diet, in which vegetables, fruits, and soy are consumed, along with some dairy products but not meat, fish, or foul. Consistent with these findings are very low isoflavone levels in predominantly carnivorous (meat-eating) individuals. Furthermore, Asian immigrants in Hawaii have a significant decrease in isoflavone levels as a consequence of changing from an Asian (soy-containing) diet to a Western diet.

Phytoestrogens are quite plentiful in the diet. There are many compounds in the diet, with diverse chemical structure, that are known to be estrogenic or antiestrogenic and that are capable of interfering with the binding of estrogen to receptor sites in the cells. Soybeans contain the principal isoflavones, genistein and daidzein, but soy sprouts also contain coumestrol, a compound that is not found to any great extent in other soy foods.

THERE IS STILL MORE TO LEARN

The mechanism of action of estrogenic compounds is quite controversial, and more research is needed to clarify these actions. Remember that estrogens are steroid molecules that are able to gain access to the cells. It seems likely that phytoestrogens induce different structural effects on the binding domains. Although phytoestrogens may work in many ways in a similar manner to naturally occurring animal estrogens, other effects may operate. Additional research is required to define the other biological effects of phytoestrogens at the cellular level.

On occasion, estrogens have been referred to as a double-edged sword. On the one hand, the beneficial effects of estrogens are clear in certain situations, such as their ability to prevent or treat osteoporosis and breast and prostate cancer. On the other hand, there are well-described adverse effects of estrogens. For example, a potent synthetic estrogen (diethylstilbestrol) is a known carcinogen, capable of crossing the placenta. Tamoxifen, an anti-estrogen, has untoward effects on stimulating the growth of cells of the lining (luminal epithelium) of the uterus. In contrast, the compound equol, which is a metabolite of phytoestrogens, does not stimulate the growth of the lining of the uterus. The circumstances of the effects of estrogen on tissues and factors that modulate the effect are very complex and not fully understood.

While this information may seem complex and perplexing, it is easier to understand when you realize that the terms "estrogenic" or "antiestrogenic" are inadequate when describing the actions of phytoestrogens. Much more scientific investigation is necessary before the agonistic or antagonistic effects of estrogen are known and the safety of phytoestrogens is more fully defined. However, it should be emphasized that no toxicity of soy isoflavones in humans, at dosage levels that are commensurate with what are consumed in soy-rich diets, is known. Further, soy isoflavones have never been associated with cancer development in animals or humans.

WHY THE DEBATE CONTINUES

Much of the safety of soy-based diets containing isoflavones may stem from misinterpretation of scientific data or unscientific reactions to "stories." For example, a toxicologist in New Zealand fed his parrots a soy-based formula, and they died. He blamed soy for their death, but failed to recognize that soy is not an approved diet for parrots. However, bad news travels fast, and this toxicologist encouraged a colleague to compile data on antinutrients contained in soy. William Shurtleff, president of the Soyfoods Center, has said, "There is not one human study demonstrating any kind of toxicity in response to soy consumption, and people have been eating soyfoods in the U.S. for decades and in Asia for hundreds of years." The report by the toxicologist and his colleague is what Shurtleff calls a "classic example of a little knowledge being dangerous."

Inevitably, some of the controversies have become political. One area in which soy-based diets appear to have been heavily criticized is their application as a protein source for bodybuilders. One popular author (S. Liebowitz) of articles that advise bodybuilders has stated, ". . . the soy protein controversy is a direct consequence of the premeditated and intentional use of confusion as a weapon; it is a coordinated campaign that is conducted (and funded) by those who sell soy products." Making statements such as this is not the best way to sort out the science and, instead, contributes to further politicizing nutritional advances.

The statements of Liebowitz and others are important in terms of being typical examples of illogical interpretation of data. This lack of logic may plague the recognition of the health benefits of soy. Controversies in the bodybuilding literature center around the effects of soy isoflavones, comparisons of the protein value between soy and eggs or whey, and some misinterpretation of the importance of cholesterol in disease states.

A 1995 editorial in *Lancet* is used by some as evidence that phytoestrogens may cause reproductive abnormalities in males. At best, this editorial suggests a tenuous link, without any documented evidence of adverse effects of soy on reproductive health. In 1995, A. Bullock, writing in the *Medical Tribune*, emphatically stated that there is clear evidence that isoflavones do not cause male reproductive problems.

Unfortunately, the arguments about the quality of soy protein are never ending. However, clear evidence exists that soy protein is an all-vegetable, cholesterol-free, high-quality protein source with virtually no fat. Like other proteins, soy has met the standard defined as generally recognized as safe as proposed by regulatory authorities such as the FDA. Soy protein meets— or often exceeds—the essential amino acid requirements established by the Food and Nutrition Board of the National Research Council and the National Academy of Sciences.

Throughout this book, you have read about the value of soy proteins. These proteins are presented in most soy foods in a format that is at least as digestible as protein derived from milk, fish, eggs, or meat, and they are of great value for nutrition and health promotion in children and adults. The addition of soy protein in the diet of Westerners has the potential to help prevent the array of diseases and disorders discussed in the chapters of this book. It can be said with confidence that soy-based diets are safe and provide powerful health benefits. Continuing debate about what is already known serves only to deprive the general public of the assurance they need in order to avail themselves the array of valuable soy foods and nutritional supplements.

The agents in soy diets that are primarily responsible for many of the health benefits are the isoflavones, particularly genistein. Usually it is the estrogenic (or antiestrogenic) effects of genistein and other isoflavones that have driven the debate. However, the discovery, more than a decade ago, of genistein in soybeans as a naturally occurring protein kinase inhibitor was a major breakthrough in medicine. This breakthrough has been grossly underestimated, and its significance was not very well explained to the general public.

THE GLOBAL VIEW SAYS IT ALL

Many hundreds of scientific studies have been reported in peer-reviewed literature that show the versatility of soy isoflavones in protecting against many diseases, including osteoporosis, coronary artery disease, and cancer. In 1995, Dr. Stephen Barnes summed up the knowledge about genistein with the following statement: "Since one-third of this planet's population consume substantial amounts of soy (and hence, genistein) and have low rates of breast and prostate cancer and of cardiovascular disease, it can be concluded that in humans, genistein is not toxic and indeed may be the direct cause of the lowered risk of these diseases. Emerging data from animal models suggest that this may be soy."

Dr. Barnes and others do not necessarily support the development of specific genistein nutritional supplements, but this is a different issue. The point is, Barnes and others recognize that consuming genistein from soy foods in the diet is safe and advantageous.

Global Health and Science

Americans spend more than 60 billion dollars per year on prescription medications. Unfortunately, this investment has not had a major effect on several life-threatening conditions that continue to compromise quality of life and lead to premature death. As you have seen, one group of these diseases, the cardiovascular disorders, begins in childhood. Given the pervasive nature of fast foods and other foods high in saturated fats, it takes a conscious effort to consume a more healthful diet containing soy and other vegetable proteins.

What should help convince you that soy foods, and plant-based diets in general, are the more healthful approach is the fact that the same degenerative diseases that affect the West are emerging in Asia and other parts of world where animal protein consumption is increasing. Rather than debating the safety of soy, perhaps we should be spending our time debating the wisdom of exporting components of a diet high in refined foods that contain considerable amounts of saturated fat to nations that have traditional diets that are healthier than ours. In the short-term, exporting fast foods (and other foods products that do not promote health) brings profits and gives the impression that the world is indeed becoming a "global village." However, when viewed over the long-run, the health consequences may be devastating for humankind. Short-term economic interests are taking precedence over improving the health of the world's population. While you may not be able to change this economic trend, you have the power to change your own diet.

Over several centuries soy has shown itself to be one of the most important, healthful, and safe foods on our planet. While research should—and indeed, must—continue to discover all the health-promoting properties of soy, Western populations can begin taking advantage of what is already known about soy. Because of the overwhelming evidence that exists, they can feel confident that they will suffer no adverse health effects from consuming well-prepared soy foods in their diets. In addition, the judicious use of dietary supplements made from soy such as soy protein isolates, soy isoflavones, and soy fiber in appropriate amounts is a safe practice in many circumstances, particularly when used with the guidance of a qualified health-care provider. I may change my mind when soy foods can be produced in an economical way and when they are "engineered" by food technologists to contain standardized amounts of the known health-giving fractions of soy. This circumstance will take time, and I reject, with a measure of vehemence, that dietary supplements made from soy are unsafe or do not play a role in promoting well-being. Let us face facts. We are unlikely to change the food preferences of Western society overnight, and the age of nutritional intervention with measured amounts of nutrients is upon us. Soy is the quintessential substrate for health-giving dietary food supplements and foods.

CHAPTER 17

The Champions of Soy and Health

The soybean has been used as a staple food in Asia for thousands of years, and its medicinal and nutritional values are deeply rooted in traditional Chinese medicine and herbalism. In 1939, Kloss stated, "A knowledge of the value of the soybean here in America is one of the greatest things that was ever launched in the food line in the history of the nation, and at this time of great poverty, want and disease, it is the most important thing that could be given to the people."

Soybeans are complete vegetable substitutes for meat, eggs, and milk, and they are easy to grow in many climates. Soybeans contain little fat, ideal amounts of protein, fiber, and a balanced mineral content with a good vitamin profile. The benefit of soy food incorporation into the diet speaks for itself.

However, I would like to trace the efforts and dedication of some individuals who have championed the cause of soy diets. Their voices are at last beginning to be heard, and they have powerful messages that are worthy of attention. Where possible, I have interviewed or interacted with these "modern day champions" of soy-based diets.

CHAI-WON CHUNG, M.D.

Dr. Chung is a pediatrician who has spent more than sixty years committed to the development of soy foods with health benefits. Over the past thirty years, he has performed much animal research to develop high quality soy milk, primarily to solve the problem of milk and lactose intolerance that is very common in infants in Korea. Dr. Chung is responsible for correcting the health of a nation with his important work.

T.W. KWON, PH.D.

T.W. Kwon is the Professor and Director of the Food Science Institute of Inje University in Korea. He is founder of the Korean Soyfood Association and has written multiple articles and books on the processing and health benefits of soy foods. Professor Kwon's forty years of excellent work on the soybean is one of the most important contributions to soy food research in the world.

MARK MESSINA, PH.D.

Mark Messina, Ph.D., is one of the world's foremost authorities on soy foods and their role in disease prevention. He is a nutritional scientist who studied at the University of Michigan and worked in the diet and cancer branch of the National Cancer Institute (NCI). His most notable achievements have been in the field of soy-based diets for cancer prevention, and he has published widely on this subject. Messina has consulted with the soybean industry for many years and has chaired several symposia and lectured widely on the health benefits of soy.

Mark Messina organized a milestone symposium on the role of soy in preventing cancer, held at the NCI in 1990. Following this workshop, the NCI launched a three million dollar research program on soy and cancer. Even more important the meeting alerted the scientific community to the potential health benefits of soy, and research on soy and cancer took off in an exponential manner afterward.

In 1994, he and his colleagues organized the First International Symposium on the Role of Soy in Preventing and Treating Chronic Disease, held in Mesa, Arizona. Thirty-four papers were presented in such categories as soy intake and cholesterol reduction, soy and heart disease prevention, and soy in the prevention of cancer. Emerging from this meeting was a clear body of evidence to support the use of soy diets or soy supplementation of the diet in the prevention of a wide variety of chronic disorders. Most notable was the focus of the meeting on the important properties of soy isoflavones, especially genistein as an example of a dietary phytoestrogen with anticancer, antiangiogenic, and other health effects.

The Second International Symposium on the Role of Soy in Preventing and Treating Chronic Disease was held in 1995, pointing to the large body of research and evidence on the role of soy in the promotion of cardiovascular wellness and cancer prevention.

Mark's book, written with his wife Virginia, *The Simple Soybean and Your Health*, is an abundant source of practical methods for the incorporation of soybeans into a Western diet. One of its most important messages is that a complete change from a Western diet to a traditional soy-based Asian diet may not be necessary to enjoy the health benefits of soybeans. He subscribes to the notion that dietary supplementation with soybean products in relatively modest amounts may be beneficial to health, claiming that nowhere is this more obvious than in the use of soy protein isolates containing isoflavones to reduce cholesterol and promote cardiovascular wellness.

WILLIAM SHURTLEFF

William Shurtleff has made countless major contributions toward informing the world of the nutritional and health benefits of soybeans. Shurtleff and his wife, Akiki Aoyagi Shurtleff, started full-time research on soy food more than twenty years ago. Their first book, *The Book of Tofu*, was an enormous success, and it is now in its second edition. It is a widely acclaimed, best-selling treatise on the nutritional power of soy in a tofu format. The book is notable in its practical advice on tofu manufacture and incorporation into the diet, with special emphasis on the protein value of soy as a solution to world nutritional needs.

Mr. Shurtleff is the president of the Soyfoods Center (P.O. Box 234, Lafayette, California, 94549-0234), which was founded in 1976. The Soyfoods Center is one of the world's leading sources of books and computerized information related to soy foods. Mr. Shurtleff's contributions to the soy food literature is voluminous and of extremely high quality. He has unique qualifications in engineering, humanities, and education from Stanford University. His academic attributes, together with his world-wide experience, have permitted the Shurtleffs to present a global view of both traditional and contemporary knowledge about soy foods. William Shurtleff must be admired as a true pioneer, with a focus on assisting in the alleviation of world hunger and disease prevention through the promotion of soy foods as healthful dietary staples.

KENNETH D.R. SETCHELL, PH.D.

Dr. Setchell is to be credited with some of the most important findings on the biological effects of isoflavones in mammals. He has a Ph.D. in steroid biochemistry, and his elegant laboratory work has done a great deal to define the importance of isoflavones (genistein and daidzein) in cancer prevention.

Setchell reports with Messina and Barnes on the overwhelming in vitro (laboratory) and in vivo (human and animal trials) data that support the beneficial role of soy isoflavones in cancer prevention. In a classic article published more than a decade ago, Setchell et al. discuss nonsteroidal estrogens of dietary origin (isoflavones) and their possible role in hormone-dependent diseases. Many of his early hypotheses have been proven in recent research, showing that isoflavones have a clear application in the prevention and perhaps treatment of cancer of diverse types.

Although soy diets have not been shown to unequivocally cure or prevent cancer completely, the supportive evidence to justify their further study is clear. The soy pathway to health can be taken with the knowledge that it is a safe option. Setchell's work on the biopharmaceutical effects of isoflavones in soy is of extreme importance.

EARL MINDELL, R.PH., PH.D.

Earl Mindell requires no introduction to anyone who is interested in using nutritional methods to promote health. In his book *The Food Medicine Bible* (1994), Dr. Mindell gives us more than an inkling of his great belief in the nutritional and health-promoting benefits of soy. This belief then became fully apparent in his later book, Earl Mindell's *Soy Miracle* (1995), in which the importance of isoflavones in disease prevention and potential cure of disease is highlighted in a highly readable, non-technical manner for the layperson.

It is notable that Mindell's interest in soybeans developed as a consequence of his interest in longevity among certain groups of Japanese people. His proposal, which I share, is that the key to the longevity of the Japanese is their lifetime consumption of soy foods. Mindell attributes much of the health benefit of soybeans to their isoflavone content (genistein and daidzein). Dr. Mindell has formulated a group of products based on soy that are promoted for fat loss, body sculpting, vibrant energy, and optimal health.

DONALD F. OTHMER

Donald F. Othmer is mentioned because he exerted a major influence on fueling my interest in soy-based diets. He was a chemical engineer of world repute, who made some of the most important contributions to the large-scale manufacture of pharmaceuticals. Following World War II, Othmer spent considerable time in the Far East advising governments on chemical manufacturing processes. During his regular trips to Japan, he recognized the health benefits of soy and developed a special interest in lecithin, which can be derived from soybeans. Othmer has told me repeatedly that he believes that soy-based diets are a key to longevity. Othmer's fame is often restricted to his major contributions to chemical engineering, but his interest in nutrition was a pivotal stimulus for me. Dr. Othmer died in 1996.

ROBERT ATKINS, M.D.

Dr. Atkins, of the Atkins Center in New York, is an alternative and contemporary health care physician par excellence. In an interview, he expressed to me his great belief in vegetable alternatives to high-carbohydrate, high-protein diets. Atkins has recognized the importance of soy-based diets in his practice and has done much to assess the literature on their health role in his valuable writings and lectures.

E.C. HENLEY

Seldom do individuals in the food industry obtain just recognition. Ms. Henley is a scientific executive with the Ralston Purina Company in St. Louis, Missouri, who has compiled a tremendous database on the health benefits of soy and applied her knowledge to inventing new ways of incorporating soy into the diet. She has proposed her thoughts on the ideal beverage for the health-conscious woman, which is based on soy products. Ms. Henley believes that soy protein isolates containing isoflavones have major potential health benefits. Protein from soy contains an amino acid profile that is highly desirable for the active woman. Soybeans are relatively low in calories, and their isoflavone content is of special importance for women, according to Ms. Henley. She is very impressed with the cholesterol-lowering potential of soy protein isolates containing isoflavones, and she believes that calcium fortification of soy protein may assist in osteoporosis prevention. Of course, Ms. Henley is highly cognizant and supportive of a potential cancer prevention role of isoflavones, especially for breast cancer.

JAMES ANDERSON, M.D.

Dr. Anderson is a physician and researcher at the University of Kentucky who is known for his work on the health benefits of dietary fiber. However, Dr. Anderson is now enjoying worldwide recognition for his groundbreaking studies on the effects of soy protein intake on serum lipids (cholesterol) published in the *New England Journal of Medicine* on August 3, 1995.

Dr. Anderson accepted the premise that diets based on vegetable protein are associated with lower risk of coronary artery disease than animal protein diets. He made a statistical review of 38 clinical trials that examined the effects of soy protein on serum cholesterol and presented a special statistical analysis of these studies. Anderson et al. were able to conclude unequivocally that "the consumption of soy protein rather than animal protein significantly decreased serum concentrations of total cholesterol, LDL cholesterol, and triglycerides." They thought that soy estrogens (isoflavones, such as genistein and daidzein) were most likely to be responsible for the cholesterol-lowering effects of soy protein.

The importance of the 1995 study by Anderson et al. is not to be minimized because these scientific observations provide a clear basis for the labeling of dietary supplements containing soy protein and isoflavones. It can be stated that soy protein isolates containing isoflavones (greater than 2 mg/gram) lower blood cholesterol and, by inference, promote cardiovascular health.

CATHY READ

Ms. Read has written a magnificent book, *Preventing Breast Cancer, The Politics of an Epidemic* (1995). In this powerful and provocative book, she stresses the medical and political inertia undermining efforts for the effective prevention of this common cancer in women. She points out that conventional medicine has failed to find a cure for breast cancer and makes a compelling argument that the root causes of breast cancer, such as diet, environment, and social structures, are amenable to correction.

In the chapter on diet and breast cancer, Ms. Read discusses the obvious role of the isoflavones in soy protein in breast cancer prevention. She states: "Soy is a particularly rich source of isoflavones and traditional Far Eastern diets are rich in soy products such as beans, tofu, miso and soy milk. The scientific evidence suggests that protective effect of a diet high in soy proteins may at least partly explain the low rates of breast cancer in China and Japan."

The value of Ms. Read's book is the practical way in which she recommends preventing breast cancer by carefully analyzing valid scientific data. Soy is one of many approaches she recommends in dietary adjustments to prevent breast cancer.

CONCLUSION

I apologize to those many other individuals who have played major and significant roles in defining the health benefits of soy. Many other people deserve an accolade for their work—the contributions are vast in number.

Suggested Reading

Akers, Keith. *A Vegetarian Sourcebook*. New York: G.P. Putnam's Sons, 1983.

Atwood, Charles. *Dr. Atwood's Low-Fat Prescription for Kids*. New York: Penguin, 1995.

Downes, John. *Soy Source*. Garden City, NY: Avery, 1989.

Editors, *Prevention Magazine*. *The Complete Book of Natural and Medicinal Cures*. Berkley, New York: Prevention Magazine Health Books, 1996.

Erasmus, Udo. *Fats That Heal, Fats that Kill*. BC: Burnaby, 1993.

Gaby, Alan. *Preventing and Reversing Osteoporosis*. Rocklin, CA: Prima Publishing, 1994.

Holt, Stephen. *The Lifestyle Commandments*, New Canaan, CT: Avery, 1998.

—— *Miracle Herbs*. New York: Carol Publishing, 1998.

—— *Soya For Health*. Larchmont, NY: Mary Ann Liebert, Inc., 1996.

Jacobi, Dana. *Soy!* Rocklin, CA: Prima, 1996.

Lappe, Frances Moore. *Diet for a Small Planet*. New York: Ballantine, 1975.

Lee, John. *What Your Doctor May Not Tell You About Menopause*. New York: Warner Books, 1996.

Love, Susan. *Dr. Susan Love's Hormone Book*. New York: Random House, 1997.

Martens, Richard, and Sherlyn Martens. *The Milk Sugar Dilemma*. Medi-Ed, 1987.

McCully, Kilmer. *The Homocysteine Revolution*. New Canaan, CT: Keats, 1997.

Messina, Mark, and Virginia Messina. *The Simple Soybean and Your Health*. NY: Avery, Garden City Park, 1994.

Mindell, Earl. *The Food Medicine Bible*. London: Souvenir Press, 1994

——*Earl Mindell's Soy Miracle*. New York: Fireside, 1995.

Ornish, Dean. *Dr. Dean Ornish's Program for Reversing Heart Disease*. New York: Ballantine, 1996.

Paino, John, and Lisa Messinger. *The Tofu Book: The New American Cuisine*. NY: Avery, Garden City, 1991.

Paish, Wilf. *Diet and Sport*. London: A and C Publishers, Ltd., 1997.

Read, Cathy. *Preventing Breast Cancer: The Politics of an Epidemic*. London, UK: Pandora, 1995.

Robbins, John. *Diet For a New America*. Walpole, NH: Stillpoint, 1987.

Schachter, Michael. *The Natural Way to a Healthy Prostate*. New Canaan, CT: Keats, 1995.

Schwarzenegger, Arnold. *Arnold's Body Building for Men*. New York: Carol Publishing, 1991.

Shandler, Nina. *Estrogen: The Natural Way*. New York: Villard, 1997.

Shurtleff, William, and Akiko Aoyagi. *The Book of Tofu*. Berkley, CA: Ten Speed Press, 1983.

Winter, Ruth. *A Consumer's Guide to Medicines in Food*. New York: Crown, 1995.

Resources and Information

The Soy Information Department
Biotherapies, Inc.
9 Commerce Rd.
Fairfield, NJ 07004
Fax line: 973-276-0639
800-700-7325

The Soyfoods Center
P.O. Box 234
Lafayette, CA 94549-0234
510-283-2991

American Soybean Association
540 Maryville Centre Drive, #390
Box 419200
St. Louis, MO 63141-9200
800-TALK SOY

Soyfoods Association of America
1 Sutter St., #300
San Francisco, CA 94104
415-939-9697

Index